Blueprints **Notes & Cases**
Biochemistry, Genetics, and Embryology

Blueprints Notes & Cases
Series Editor: Aaron B. Caughey MD, MPP, MPH

Blueprints *Notes & Cases—Microbiology and Immunology*
Monica Gandhi, Paul Baum, C. Bradley Hare, Aaron B. Caughey

Blueprints *Notes & Cases—Biochemistry, Genetics, and Embryology*
Juan E. Vargas, Aaron B. Caughey, Annie Tan, Jonathan Z. Li

Blueprints *Notes & Cases—Pharmacology*
Katherine Y. Yang, Larissa R. Graff, Aaron B. Caughey

Blueprints *Notes & Cases—Pathophysiology: Cardiovascular, Endocrine, and Reproduction*
Gordon Leung, Susan H. Tran, Tina O. Tan, Aaron B. Caughey

Blueprints *Notes & Cases—Pathophysiology: Pulmonary, Gastrointestinal, and Rheumatology*
Michael Filbin, Lisa M. Lee, Brian L. Shaffer, Aaron B. Caughey

Blueprints *Notes & Cases—Pathophysiology: Renal, Hematology, and Oncology*
Aaron B. Caughey, Christie del Castillo, Nancy Palmer, Karen Spizer, Dana N. Tuttle

Blueprints *Notes & Cases—Neuroscience*
Robert T. Wechsler, Alexander M. Morss, Courtney J. Wusthoff, Aaron B. Caughey

Blueprints *Notes & Cases—Behavioral Science and Epidemiology*
Judith Neugroschl, Jennifer Hoblyn, Christie del Castillo, Aaron B. Caughey

Blueprints **Notes & Cases**
Biochemistry, Genetics, and Embryology

Juan E. Vargas, MD
Acting Chief of Obstetrics
San Francisco General Hospital
Department of Obstetrics, Gynecology, and Reproductive Sciences
University of California, San Francisco
San Francisco, California

Aaron B. Caughey, MD, MPP, MPH
Clinical Instructor in Maternal-Fetal Medicine
Department of Obstetrics and Gynecology
University of California, San Francisco
San Francisco, California
Doctoral Candidate, Health Services and Policy Analysis
University of California, Berkeley
Berkeley, California

Annie Tan, MD, PhD
Resident
Department of Obstetrics & Gynecology
University of California, San Francisco
San Francisco, California

Jonathan Z. Li
Class of 2003
University of California, San Francisco School of Medicine
San Francisco, California

Series Editor: Aaron B. Caughey, MD, MPP, MPH

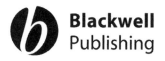

Blackwell
Publishing

Blackwell Publishing, Inc., 350 Main Street, Malden, Massachusetts 02148-5018, USA
Blackwell Publishing Ltd, 9600 Garsington Road, Oxford OX4 2DQ, UK
Blackwell Science Asia Pty Ltd, 550 Swanston Street, Carlton, Victoria 3053, Australia

04 05 06 07 5 4 3 2 1

ISBN: 1–4051-0354-X

Library of Congress Cataloging-in-Publication Data

Biochemistry, genetics, and embryology / Juan E. Vargas . . . [et al.]. — 1st ed.
    p. ; cm. — (Blueprints notes & cases)
  Includes index.
  ISBN 1-4051-0354-X
  1. Clinical biochemistry—Case studies. 2. Medical genetics—Case studies. 3. Embryology—Case studies. I. Vargas, Juan E. II. Series.
  [DNLM: 1. Biochemistry—Problems and Exercises. 2. Embryology—Problems and Exercises. 3. Genetics—Problems and Exercises. QU 18.2 B6147 2004]
  RB112.5.B555 2004
  612'.015—dc21
                                                               2003007072

A catalogue record for this title is available from the British Library

Acquisitions: Beverly Copland
Development: Julia Casson
Production: Jennifer Kowalewski
Cover design: Hannus Design Associates
Interior design: Janet Bollow Associates
Typesetter: Peirce Graphic Services, in Stuart, Florida
Printed and bound by Courier Companies, in Westford, MA

For further information on Blackwell Publishing, visit our website: www.blackwellpublishing.com

Notice: The indications and dosages of all drugs in this book have been recommended in the medical literature and conform to the practices of the general community. The medications described do not necessarily have specific approval by the Food and Drug Administration for use in the diseases and dosages for which they are recommended. The package insert for each drug should be consulted for use and dosage as approved by the FDA. Because standards for usage change, it is advisable to keep abreast of revised recommendations, particularly those concerning new drugs.

Contents

I. BIOCHEMISTRY

II. GENETICS

III. EMBRYOLOGY

Contributors

Kimberly Gibson, M.D.
Resident in Obstetrics and Gynecology
Kaiser Permanente
San Francisco, CA

Holbrook Kohrt
Class of 2004
Stanford Medical School
Palo Alto, CA

Elaine Yu
Class of 2004
University of California, San Francisco Medical School
San Francisco, CA

Eric Kenley
Class of 2004
University of California, San Francisco Medical School
San Francisco, CA

Reviewers

Preface

The first two years of medical school are a demanding time for medical students. Whether the school follows a traditional curriculum or one that is case-based, every student is expected to learn and be able to apply basic science information in a clinical situation.

Medical schools are increasingly using clinical presentations as the background to teach the basic sciences. Case-based learning has become more common at many medical schools as it offers a way to catalogue the multitude of symptoms, syndromes and diseases in medicine.

Blueprints Notes & Cases is a new series by Blackwell Publishing designed to provide students a textbook to study the basic science topics combined with clinical data. This method of learning is also the way to prepare for the clinical case format of USMLE questions. The eight books in this series will make the basic science topics not only more interesting, but also more meaningful and memorable. Students will be learning not only the why of a principle, but also how it might commonly be seen in practice.

The books in the *Blueprints* Notes & Cases series feature a comprehensive collection of cases which are designed to introduce one or more basic science topics. Through these cases, students gain an understanding of the coursework as they learn to:

- Think through the cases
- Look for classic presentations of most common diseases and syndromes
- Integrate the basic science content with clinical application
- Prepare for course exams and Step 1 USMLE
- Be prepared for clinical rotations

This series covers all the essential material needed in the basic science courses. Where possible, the books are organized in an organ-based system.

Clinical cases lead off and are the basis for discussion of the basic science content. A list of "**thought questions**" follows the case presentation. These questions are designed to challenge the reader to begin to think about how basic science topics apply to real-life clinical situations. The **answers to these questions** are integrated within the **basic science review and discussion** that follows. This offers a clinical framework from which to understand the basic content.

The discussion section is followed by a high-yield **Thumbnail table and Key Points box** which highlight and summarize the essential information presented in the discussion.

The cases also include two to four **multiple-choice questions** that allow readers to check their knowledge of that topic. Many of the answer explanations provide an opportunity for further discussion by delving into more depth in related areas. An **answer key** for these questions is at the end of the section for easy reference, and **full answer explanations** can be found at the end of the book.

This new series was designed to provide comprehensive content in a concise and templated format for ease in learning. A dedicated attempt was made to include sufficient art, tables, and clinical treatment, all while keeping the books from becoming too lengthy. We know you have much to read and that what you want is high-yield, vital facts.

The authors and series editor for these eight books, as well as everyone in editorial, production, sales and marketing at Blackwell Publishing, have worked long and hard to provide new textbooks to help you learn and be able to apply what you've learned. We engaged in multiple student email surveys and many focus groups to "hear what you needed" in new basic science level textbooks to meet the current curriculums, tests, and coursework. We know that you value this "student to student" approach, and sincerely hope you like what we have put together **just for you.**

Blackwell Publishing and the authors wish you success in your studies and your future medical career. Please feel free to offer us any comments or suggestions on these new books at blue@bos.blackwellpublishing.com.

Acknowledgments

To Pia and Edmundo, for their never ending encouragement and support. To Javier, Ale, and Andrés, my pride and joy. And to Holly, my companion and friend on this long exciting journey.
Juan

To my parents, Bill and Carol, thank you for all of your support over the years. To my mentors Drs. Washington, Norton, Kuppermann, Sandberg, Lieberman, and Shipp and Professors Robinson, Rabin, Hu, and Luft: I promise I will focus a bit more. Finally, to my wife, Susan, thank you for your support, advice, and patience.
Aaron

To my best friend and husband, Richard, for all his love, support, and encouragement.
Annie

To my mother and father. You have given me life, love, and a passion for learning. Thanks for everything.
Jon

Abbreviations

7-DHC	7-dehydrocholesterol	CoA	coenzyme A
AA	arachidonic acid	CO	carbon monoxide
ACAT	acyl-CoA:cholesterol acyl transferase	CO_2	carbon dioxide
ACTH	adrenocorticotropic hormone	CPS	carbamoylphosphate synthetase
ACP	acyl carrier protein	CT	computed tomography
ADA	adenosine deaminase	CVS	chorionic villus sampling
AD	autosomal dominant	D&C	dilation and curettage
ADP	adenosine diphosphate	DES	diethylstilbestrol
AFP	alpha-fetoprotein	DHF	dihydrofolate
AIP	acute intermittent porphyria	DNA	deoxyribonucleic acid
ALA	aminolevulinic acid	DS	Down syndrome
AMP	adenosine monophosphate	dsDNA	double-stranded DNA
ANS	autonomic nervous system	dTMP	deoxythymidine monophosphate
APKD	adult polycystic kidney disease	DTRs	deep tendon reflexes
AR	autosomal recessive	dUMP	deoxyuridine monophosphate
ASD	atrial septal defect	ED	emergency department
A-T	ataxia-telangiectasia	ECG	electrocardiogram
ATM	ataxia-telangiectasia mutated gene	ELISA	enzyme-linked immunosorbent assay
ATP	adenosine triphosphate	ETC	electron transport chain
BP	blood pressure	$FADH_2$	flavin adenine dinucleotide (reduced)
BPG-2,3	bisphosphoglycerate	FAE	fetal alcohol effect
BRA	bilateral renal agenesis	FAS	fetal alcohol syndrome
CAH	congenital adrenal hyperplasia	FGFR	fibroblast growth factor receptor
cAMP	cyclic AMP	FISH	fluorescent in situ hybridization
CBC	complete blood count	G0	gap 0
CBS	cystathionine β-synthase	G1	gap 1
CD4	CD4$^+$ cell count	G2	gap 2
CDH	congenital diaphragmatic hernia	G6P	glucose 6-phosphate
Cdk	cyclin-dependent kinase	G6PD	glucose-6-phosphate dehydrogenase
CF	cystic fibrosis	GA	gestational age
CFTR	cystic fibrosis transmembrane regulator	GALT	galactose 1-uridyltransferase
CHD	congenital heart disease	G_i	inhibitory G protein
CMP	cytidylate	GI	gastrointestinal tract
CMV	cytomegalovirus	GMP	guanosine monophosphate
CN	cranial nerve	G_s	stimulatory G protein
CNS	central nervous system	GTD	gestational trophoblastic disease

GTP	guanosine triphosphate		mRNA	messenger RNA
GxPy	gravida x para y		MSAFP	maternal serum alpha-fetoprotein
hCG	human chorionic gonadotropin		mtDNA	mitochondrial DNA
Hgb	hemoglobin		MTHFR	methylenetetrahydrofolate reductase
HDL	high-density lipoprotein		NADH	nicotinamide adenine dinucleotide, reduced
HEENT	head, eyes, ears, nose, throat		NADPH	nicotinamide adenine dinucleotide phosphate, reduced
Hex A	hexosaminidase A		NF	neurofibromatosis
HIV	human immunodeficiency virus		NF1	neurofibromatosis type 1
HLA	human leukocyte antigen		NF2	neurofibromatosis type 2
HMG-CoA	hydroxymethylglutaryl-CoA		NS	normal saline
HNPCC	hereditary nonpolyposis colon cancer		NSAIDs	nonsteroidal anti-inflammatory drugs
HR	heart rate		NSVD	normal spontaneous vaginal delivery
HSV	herpes simplex virus		NTD	neural tube defect
HTLV	human t-cell lymphotropic virus		O_2	oxygen
IDL	intermediate-density lipoprotein		O_2 Sat	oxygen saturation
IEM	inborn error of metabolism		OI	osteogenesis imperfecta
IMP	inosine monophosphate		PAH	phenylalanine hydroxylase
IQ	intelligence quotient		PBG	porphobilinogen
IRS	insulin receptor substrate		PCP	primary care provider
IV	intravenous		PCP	*Pneumocystis carinii* pneumonia
IVF	in vitro fertilization		PCR	polymerase chain reaction
IVIG	intravenous immune globulin		PDA	patent ductus arteriosus
LCAT	lecithin-cholesterol acyltransferase		PEP	phosphoenolpyruvate
LDL	low-density lipoprotein		PFK	phosphofructokinase
LHON	Leber's hereditary optic neuropathy		PG	prostaglandin
LMP	last menstrual period		PGI_2	prostaglandin I_2; prostacyclin
LT	leukotriene		PK	pyruvate kinase
M	mitosis		PKU	phenylketonuria
MCAD	medium-chain acyl-CoA dehydrogenase		PNS	parasympathetic nervous system
MD	myotonic dystrophy		PRPP	5-phosphoribosyl-1-pyrophosphate
MELAS	*mitochondrial encephalopathy, lactic acidosis, and stroke-like syndrome*		PT	physical therapy
MFI	multifactorial inheritance		PTH	parathyroid hormone
MHC	major histocompatibility complex		Rb	retinoblastoma
MI	myocardial infarction		RCT	randomized controlled trials
MoM	multiples of the median		RDS	respiratory distress syndrome
MRI	magnetic resonance imaging		RFLP	restriction fragment length polymorphism

RNA	ribonucleic acid		**TMP-SMX**	trimethoprim-sulfamethoxazole
r/o	rule out		**ToRCHeS**	toxoplasmosis, rubella, CMV, herpes simplex virus, syphilis
RR	respiratory rate		**tRNA**	transfer RNA
rRNA	ribosomal RNA		**TS**	tuberous sclerosis
S	synthesis		**TSH**	thyroid-stimulating hormone
SAB	spontaneous abortion		**TSST**	toxic shock syndrome toxin
SCID	severe combined immunodeficiency		**TXA$_2$**	thromboxane A$_2$
Shh	sonic hedgehog		**UA**	urinalysis
SIDS	sudden infant death syndrome		**UCD**	urea cycle disorders
SLO	Smith-Lemli-Opitz syndrome		**UMP**	uridine monophosphate
snRNA	small nuclear RNA		**US**	ultrasound
snRNP	small ribonucleoprotein particle		**VCFS**	velocardiofacial syndrome
T	temperature		**VLDL**	very-low-density lipoprotein
TCA	tricarboxylic acid		**VSD**	ventricular septal defect
TCR	T-cell receptor		**WBCs**	white blood cells
THF	tetrahydrofolate			

Normal Ranges of Laboratory Values

BLOOD, PLASMA, SERUM

Alanine aminotransferase (ALT, GPT at 30 C)	8–20 U/L
Amylase, serum	25–125 U/L
Aspartate aminotransferase (AST, GOT at 30 C)	8–20 U/L
Bilirubin, serum (adult) Total // Direct	0.1–1.0 mg/dL // 0.0–0.3 mg/dL
Calcium, serum (Ca^{2+})	8.4–10.2 mg/dL
Cholesterol, serum	Rec: < 200 mg/dL
Cortisol, serum	0800 h: 5–23 μg/dL // 1600 h: 3–15 μg/dL
	2000 h: $\leq$ 50% of 0800 h
Creatine kinase, serum	Male: 25–90 U/L
	Female: 10–70 U/L
Creatinine, serum	0.6–1.2 mg/dL
Electrolytes, serum	
Sodium (Na^+)	136–145 mEq/L
Chloride (Cl^-)	95–105 mEq/L
Potassium (K^+)	3.5–5.0 mEq/L
Bicarbonate (HCO_3^-)	22–28 mEq/L
Magnesium (Mg^{2+})	1.5–2.0 mEq/L
Ferritin, serum	Male: 15–200 ng/mL
	Female: 12–150 ng/mL
Follicle-stimulating hormone, serum/plasma	Male: 4–25 mIU/mL
	Female: premenopause 4–30 mIU/mL
	midcycle peak 10–90 mIU/mL
	postmenopause 40–250 mIU/mL
Gases, arterial blood (room air)	
pH	7.35–7.45
P_{CO_2}	33–45 mm Hg
P_{O_2}	75–105 mm Hg
Glucose, serum	Fasting: 70–110 mg/dL
	2-h postprandial: < 120 mg/dL
Growth hormone—arginine stimulation	Fasting: < 5 ng/mL
	provocative stimuli: > 7 ng/mL
Iron	50–70 μg/dL
Lactate dehydrogenase, serum	45–90 U/L
Luteinizing hormone, serum/plasma	Male: 6–23 mIU/mL
	Female: follicular phase 5–30 mIU/mL
	midcycle 75–150 mIU/mL
	postmenopause 30–200 mIU/mL
Osmolality, serum	275–295 mOsmol/kg
Parathyroid hormone, serum, N-terminal	230–630 pg/mL
Phosphate (alkaline), serum (p-NPP at 30 C)	20–70 U/L
Phosphorus (inorganic), serum	3.0–4.5 mg/dL
Prolactin, serum (hPRL)	< 20 ng/mL
Proteins, serum	
Total (recumbent)	6.0–7.8 g/dL
Albumin	3.5–5.5 g/dL
Globulin	2.3–3.5 g/dL
Thyroid-stimulating hormone, serum or plasma	0.5–5.0 μU/mL
Thyroidal iodine (^{123}I) uptake	8–30% of administered dose/24 h
Thyroxine (T_4), serum	5–12 μg/dL
Triglycerides, serum	35–160 mg/dL
Triiodothyronine (T_3), serum (RIA)	115–190 ng/dL
Triiodothyronine (T_3), resin uptake	25–35%
Urea nitrogen, serum (BUN)	7–18 mg/dL
Uric acid, serum	3.0–8.2 mg/dL

CEREBROSPINAL FLUID

Cell count	0–5 cells/mm^3
Chloride	118–132 mEq/L
Gamma globulin	3–12% total proteins
Glucose	40–70 mg/dL
Pressure	70–180 mm H_2O
Proteins, total	< 40 mg/dL

HEMATOLOGIC

Bleeding time (template)	2–7 minutes
Erythrocyte count	Male: 4.3–5.9 million/mm^3
	Female: 3.5–5.5 million/mm^3
Erythrocyte sedimentation rate (Westergren)	Male: 0–15 mm/h
	Female: 0–20 mm/h
Hematocrit	Male: 41–53%
	Female: 36–46%
Hemoglobin A$_{1C}$	≤ 6%
Hemoglobin, blood	Male: 13.5–17.5 g/dL
	Female: 12.0–16.0 g/dL
Leukocyte count and differential	
Leukocyte count	4500–11,000/mm^3
Segmented neutrophils	54–62%
Bands	3–5%
Eosinophils	1–3%
Basophils	0–0.75%
Lymphocytes	25–33%
Monocytes	3–7%
Mean corpuscular hemoglobin	25.4–34.6 pg/cell
Mean corpuscular hemoglobin concentration	31–36% Hb/cell
Mean corpuscular volume	80–100 μm^3
Partial thromboplastin time (activated)	25–40 seconds
Platelet count	150,000–400,000/mm^3
Prothrombin time	11–15 seconds
Reticulocyte count	0.5–1.5% of red cells
Thrombin time	< 2 seconds deviation from control
Volume	
Plasma	Male: 25–43 mL/kg
	Female: 28–45 mL/kg
Red cell	Male: 20–36 mL/kg
	Female: 19–31 mL/kg

SWEAT

Chloride	0–35 mmol/L

URINE

Calcium	100–300 mg/24 h
Chloride	Varies with intake
Creatine clearance	Male: 97–137 mL/min
	Female: 88–128 mL/min
Osmolality	50–1400 mOsmol/kg
Oxalate	8–40 μg/mL
Potassium	Varies with diet
Proteins, total	< 150 mg/24 h
Sodium	Varies with diet
Uric acid	Varies with diet

Biochemistry

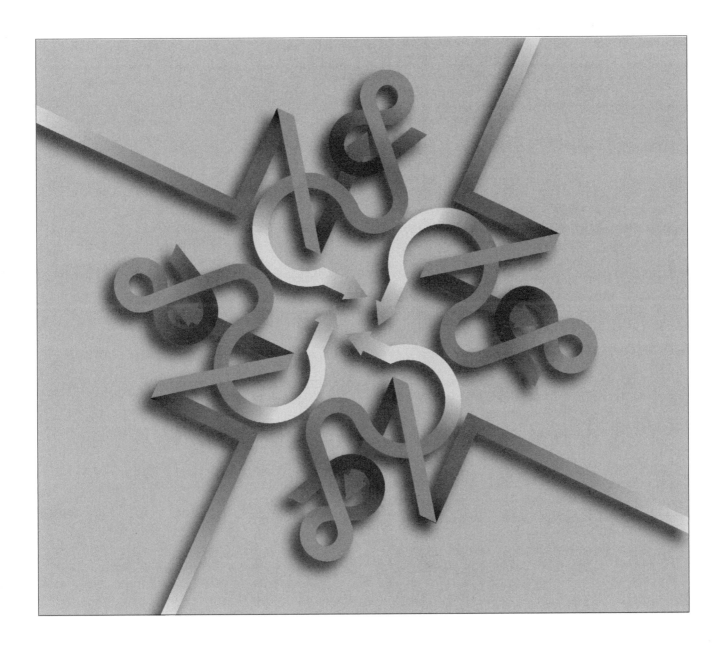

> **HPI:** HA is a 2½-year-old boy brought in for a routine visit to his pediatrician. On review of systems, his parents report that he has been increasingly fatigued over the past few months. He tires easily when playing outside and gets short of breath when roughhousing with his older brother. There has been no recent illness and he has no other significant medical history.
>
> **PE:** He is slightly tachycardic and notably pale. He has no gross jaundice but a mild scleral icterus. The exam of the lungs and heart shows no abnormalities; however, on abdominal exam, he has an enlarged spleen.
>
> **Labs:** A complete blood cell (CBC) count reveals a normocytic anemia, with a hematocrit of 23%. On inspection of the erythrocytes on peripheral smear, they are noted to be spiculated with an increase in reticulocytes.

Thought Questions

- What enzyme deficiency in glycolysis will lead to this clinical scenario most commonly?

- What other enzymes in this pathway may be deficient and lead to similar clinical outcomes?

- Why are erythrocytes particularly susceptible to pyruvate kinase (PK) deficiency?

- Why would PK deficiency lead to hemolytic anemia?

Basic Science Review and Discussion

PK is involved in the conversion of **phosphoenolpyruvate to enolpyruvate,** one of the two steps of glycolysis that generates adenosine triphosphate (ATP) by hydrolyzing a phosphate bound to the initial molecule. A review of the steps of glycolysis is shown in Figure 1-1. During glycolysis, which occurs in the cytosol, two steps require ATP: the addition of phosphate moieties by **hexokinase and phosphofructokinase** (PFK). Further on, glycolysis generates ATP during the release of phosphate by phosphoglycerate kinase and PK. Thus, it might seem that there should be an even trade-off during glycolysis, but the latter two reactions occur after glycolysis has cleaved glucose into two 3-carbon molecules, glyceraldehyde 3-phosphate and dihydroxyacetone phosphate, which are isomers. Because each of these molecules goes through the latter half of glycolysis, there is a net production of two ATP molecules from each molecule of glucose. There is also a net production of two reduced nicotinamide adenine dinucleotide **(NADH)** molecules, which will normally generate three **ATP** molecules under aerobic conditions. However, this is seen primarily in birds, which use the **malate shuttle** to move NADH to the mitochondria, whereas most mammals use the **glycerol phosphate shuttle,** which generates only two ATP molecules per NADH molecule generated in the cytosol.

Glycolysis is regulated primarily by control of PFK-1 and secondarily at hexokinase and PK. Generally, when there exists an abundance of high-energy molecules such as ATP, these enzymes' activity is decreased. Conversely, when levels of ATP are low, the activity of these enzymes is increased. When levels of ATP and citrate are high, PFK-1 is inhibited; and with accumulation of adenosine monophosphate (AMP), PFK-1 is activated. Similarly, PK is inhibited by ATP and acetyl-coenzyme A (acetyl-CoA) and activated by increased amounts of fructose 1,6-bisphosphate.

Bioenergetics The molecule **pyruvate** is the final product from glycolysis. It can undergo a variety of transformations including (1) conversion to **lactate** in the cytosol under anaerobic conditions; (2) conversion to **alanine** in the skeletal muscle; (3) conversion to **acetyl-CoA,** which enters the tricarboxylic acid (TCA) cycle and is oxidized generating NADH and reduced-form flavin adenine dinucleotide (FADH$_2$) molecules; and (4) carboxylation to **oxaloacetate,** which can be used in the TCA cycle or gluconeogenesis. If pyruvate is converted to acetyl-CoA, it generates an NADH molecule, then by undergoing oxidation in the TCA cycle under aerobic conditions, it generates three more NADH molecules, an FADH$_2$ molecule, and a guanosine triphosphate (GTP) molecule. After undergoing the electron transport chain (ETC), the net equivalent is 15 ATP molecules per each molecule of pyruvate, or 36 ATP molecules per glucose.

Pyruvate Kinase Deficiency Because glycolysis is a primary source for ATP and it generates molecules that enter the TCA cycle and ETC during aerobic conditions, decreased enzyme activity throughout glycolysis can be problematic, and dysfunctional and nonfunctional enzymes in glycolysis such as phosphoglucoisomerase, hexokinase, PFK, and others have been identified. PK deficiency is one of the more common enzymatic defects in glycolysis that has been identified and can present with a clinical spectrum. Commonly, the enzyme defect is not lethal and is most detrimental to erythrocytes because they have no mitochondria and are entirely dependent on glycolysis for the generation of ATP. The ATP is required for the erythrocytes to maintain

Glycolysis:

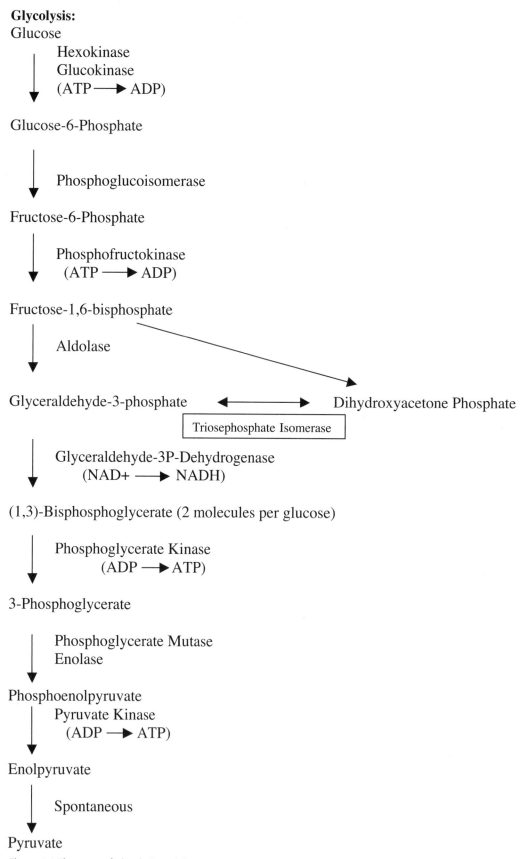

Glucose

    Hexokinase
    Glucokinase
    (ATP ⟶ ADP)

Glucose-6-Phosphate

    Phosphoglucoisomerase

Fructose-6-Phosphate

    Phosphofructokinase
    (ATP ⟶ ADP)

Fructose-1,6-bisphosphate

    Aldolase

Glyceraldehyde-3-phosphate ⟷ Dihydroxyacetone Phosphate

Triosephosphate Isomerase

    Glyceraldehyde-3P-Dehydrogenase
    (NAD+ ⟶ NADH)

(1,3)-Bisphosphoglycerate (2 molecules per glucose)

    Phosphoglycerate Kinase
    (ADP ⟶ ATP)

3-Phosphoglycerate

    Phosphoglycerate Mutase
    Enolase

Phosphoenolpyruvate

    Pyruvate Kinase
    (ADP ⟶ ATP)

Enolpyruvate

    Spontaneous

Pyruvate

Figure 1-1 The steps of glycolysis and the enzymes that catalyze these steps.

the biconcave shape. The abnormal erythrocyte shape worsens in the spleen, which is particularly anaerobic, leading to increased clearance of these cells by the spleen. Thus, patients present with hemolytic anemia of varying severity. Most commonly, patients present in early childhood with anemia, splenomegaly, and icterus. On the peripheral smear, spiculated red blood cells (RBCs) are seen with an increase in reticulocytes.

Case Conclusion   HA is given a blood transfusion, and after a lengthy discussion with his parents, the decision is made to manage him medically with daily folic acid supplementation. However, he presents with hemolytic anemia twice more in the next year and the decision is made to proceed with a splenectomy. This is effective and he maintains a normal hematocrit level over the following year.

Thumbnail: Glycolysis

Glycolysis is a series of enzymatic reactions that convert glucose under differing conditions:

Anaerobic conditions: Glucose + 2 Adenosine diphosphate (ADP) → 2 Lactate + 2 ATP

Aerobic conditions: Glucose + 2 ADP + 2 NAD$^+$ → 2 Pyruvate + 2 ATP + 2 NADH

Key Points

▶ Regulation of glycolysis is primarily maintained by inhibition of PFK-1, PK, and hexokinase, which are generally activated by a low-energy state with accumulation of AMP or precursors such as fructose-2,6-bisphosphate and inhibited by a high-energy state with accumulation of ATP or molecules such as citrate (PFK-1) or acetyl-CoA (PK).

▶ PK deficiency leads to diminished activity of glycolysis, which is particularly detrimental in RBCs, which lack mitochondria and are therefore unable to generate ATP any other way.

Questions

1. In a patient without any enzyme deficiencies who undergoes glycolysis and has normal cytosol and mitochondria, how many molecules of NADH are generated from each molecule of glucose?
    A. 4
    B. 5
    C. 6
    D. 8
    E. 10

2. In the case presented, PK deficiency leads to hemolytic anemia. However, deficiencies in other enzymes in glycolysis do not necessarily lead to hemolytic anemia. In fact, of the following enzyme deficiencies, one does not lead to hemolytic anemia. That enzyme is?
    A. Glucose-6-phosphate dehydrogenase (G6PD)
    B. Hexokinase
    C. Aldolase
    D. Pyruvate dehydrogenase
    E. Phosphoglycerate kinase

HPI: FT is a 4-month-old infant who is brought to his pediatrician because of increasing lethargy. FT has never fed well or been a particularly active baby. His parents initially thought he just constitutionally had lower energy than his older brother, but over the past several weeks, FT has become increasingly more "floppy" and has a diminishing appetite. Occasionally, his parents note that one of his extremities will extend and be stiff for a few seconds, but they have not noticed any sudden loss of consciousness or generalized seizures. FT was the product of a normal, full-term pregnancy.

PE: He has normal vital signs. He is unable to hold up his head and does not grasp a finger when placed in his hand. His suck reflex is weak. On neurologic exam, he does not noticeably follow a brightly colored toy or respond to facial expressions. His deep tendon reflexes (DTRs) are hyperactive. During the exam, you note the left leg extend, undergo several clonic movements, and then relax.

Labs: His CBC and electrolyte counts are normal, but there is an elevated anion gap and elevated lactate and pyruvate levels.

Thought Questions

- How does pyruvate enter the TCA cycle?

- Describe the steps of the pyruvate dehydrogenase complex.

- What are the key steps of the TCA cycle?

- What is the difference in bioenergetics with and without the TCA cycle?

Basic Science Review and Discussion

The end product of **glycolysis is pyruvate,** which is converted to **lactate** by **lactate dehydrogenase.** To generate more energy from glucose than glycolysis can, pyruvate must be converted to **acetyl-CoA,** which can enter the **TCA cycle.** The conversion of pyruvate to acetyl-CoA is performed by an enzymatic complex called **pyruvate dehydrogenase.**

Pyruvate Dehydrogenase **Pyruvate dehydrogenase** consists of three enzymes (**pyruvate decarboxylase** [E_1], **dihydrolipoyl transacetylase** [E_2], and **dihydrolipoyl dehydrogenase** [E_3]) and five coenzymes (flavin adenine dinucleotide [FAD], oxidized nicotinamide adenine dinucleotide [NAD^+], CoA, thiamine pyrophosphate [TPP], and lipoic acid). The C3 pyruvate molecule releases carbon dioxide (CO_2) to become a C2 molecule when interacting with E_1 and TPP. E_2, with lipoic acid and CoA, then catalyzes its oxidation and adds the CoA moiety. E_3, using the FAD and NAD^+ as coenzymes, then regenerates the lipoic acid. These three enzymes act in concert to convert pyruvate to acetyl-CoA, and the molecule is bound to the enzyme complex throughout its transformation. In addition to acetyl-CoA, an NADH molecule is generated. Of note, this NADH generates only two molecules of ATP during oxidative phosphoryla-

tion as compared with the three normally generated by NADH (Figure 2-1).

TCA Cycle The **citric acid,** or tricarboxylic acid (TCA), **cycle** is responsible for generating the bulk of ATP directly and in concert with the electron transport chain in mitochondria. The TCA cycle can be thought of as beginning when acetyl-CoA is added to oxaloacetate to form citrate. The citrate molecule then undergoes a series of reactions (see Figure 2-1) that convert it back to oxaloacetate. The result of these reactions is the production of three molecules of NADH, one $FADH_2$, and one GTP.

Bioenergetics During glycolysis, each molecule of glucose produces two pyruvate molecules, two ATP molecules, and two NADH molecules. In the conversion from pyruvate to acetyl-CoA, two more NADH molecules are generated. Then the two pyruvate molecules entering the TCA cycle generate six NADH, two $FADH_2$, and two GTP molecules. The $FADH_2$ and NADH molecules generated by two of the NADH molecules each produce two ATP molecules, and the rest produce three ATP molecules each. The net total is 36 ATP molecules per each molecule of glucose that goes through all the steps and cycles. Four of the ATP molecules are generated by substrate phosphorylation, which is directly during the metabolic pathway. The other 32 ATP molecules are created via **oxidative phosphorylation.**

Pyruvate Dehydrogenase Deficiency An enzyme deficiency of any of the three components of pyruvate dehydrogenase, E_1, E_2, or E_3, can lead to a disastrous syndrome, commonly characterized by the symptoms of FT in the case presented. Without being able to convert pyruvate to acetyl-CoA, much of the efficiency of bioenergetics is lost. In addition, a buildup of pyruvate then leads to a buildup of lactate and lactic acidosis. In addition, acetyl-CoA is used as a building block in other biochemical pathways, in particular to build fatty acids.

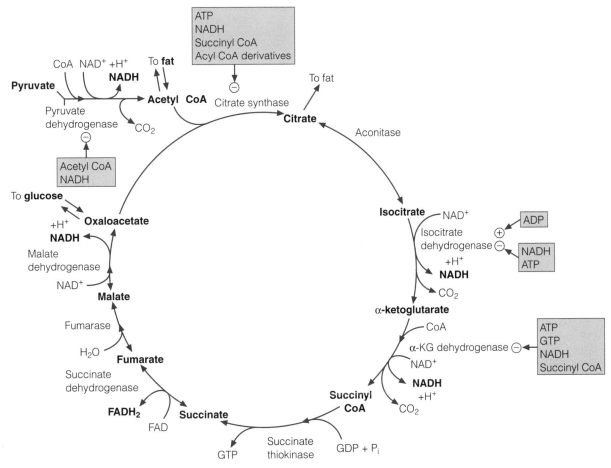

Figure 2-1 The steps of the TCA cycle. ⊖ = negative inhibition, ⊕ = positive feedback.

Case Conclusion   FT's pediatrician consults a metabolic specialist. Enzyme activity tests are done, which reveal minimal E_3 activity. The metabolic specialist recommends a high-fat, high-thiamine diet in hopes of overcoming the decreased fat production and for the thiamine to increase whatever minimal pyruvate dehydrogenase activity FT has. The dietary intervention does not seem to help and FT's signs and symptoms worsen. At age 9 months, he succumbs to his illness and dies of respiratory failure.

Thumbnail: TCA Cycle

Important Reactions in Pyruvate Dehydrogenase

1. Pyruvate + TPP $\xrightarrow{E1}$ TPP − COH − CH_3 + CO_2
2. TPP − COH − CH_3 + CoA + Lipoic acid $\xrightarrow{E2}$ Acetyl-CoA + TPP + Lipoic acid (reduced form)
3. Lipoic acid (reduced form) + NAD^+ $\xrightarrow{E3, FAD}$ Lipoic acid + NADH

Net reaction:

Pyruvate + CoA + NAD^+ $\xrightarrow{E1, E2, E3}$ Acetyl-CoA + CO_2 + NADH

Net bioenergetics in the TCA cycle:

Acetyl-CoA + 3 NAD^+ + FAD + GDP $\longrightarrow$ CoASH + 2 CO_2 + 3 NADH + $FADH_2$ + GTP

Key Points

▶ Pyruvate dehydrogenase is a three-enzyme complex that converts pyruvate to acetyl-CoA.

▶ Acetyl-CoA initially enters the TCA cycle by combining with oxaloacetate to form citric acid.

▶ The two NADH molecules formed by pyruvate dehydrogenase generate only two ATP molecules each.

▶ With an enzyme deficiency, there is a buildup of the precursor molecule and its other breakdown products (in this case, pyruvate and lactate).

Questions

1. FT, the baby who has pyruvate dehydrogenase deficiency in the presented case, undergoes an autopsy. Which of the following findings would be consistent with this syndrome?

   A. Multiple fractures
   B. Large cardiac ventricular septal defect (VSD)
   C. Enlarged liver
   D. Decreased myelination in the brain
   E. A cyst on the lateral neck

2. If a patient was missing the enzyme that catalyzes the entrance of acetyl-CoA into the TCA cycle, which of the following would most likely occur?

   A. Decreased myelination in the brain
   B. Enlarged liver
   C. Multiple fractures
   D. Elevated acetyl-CoA levels
   E. Decreased oxaloacetate levels

HPI: NS is a 9-month-old female infant who is brought to the emergency department (ED) by her parents who complain of increasingly listless behavior and decreased appetite. They are concerned that NS may have an infection, but her temperature is normal. She also has no cough, vomiting, or diarrhea. On further history, they report that NS was seemingly developing normally throughout her first 4 to 6 months of life, but she has slept more and has been less interested in eating for several months.

PE: She is a floppy baby, not holding up her head, and she has a normal ear exam but has a diminished light reflex. Both her tone and her reflexes are diminished, and she has a slightly enlarged liver.

Labs: Normal CBC count, elevated pyruvate and lactate, and profound hypoglycemia.

Thought Questions

- What is the gluconeogenesis pathway?

- How does the pathway differ from glycolysis?

- How might the body compensate for a lack of gluconeogenesis?

Basic Science Review and Discussion

Aside from digestion and absorption from the gastrointestinal (GI) tract, glucose can be generated in two ways: One is the breakdown of glycogen, and the other is to synthesize it from smaller C2, C3, and C4 molecules. Disturbances in the metabolism of glycogen can lead to several families of disorders, the glycogen storage diseases, which vary in severity. Deficiencies in gluconeogenesis tend to be more severe, which we discuss later, but first we elucidate the gluconeogenesis pathway.

Gluconeogenesis Glucose can be regenerated from its final product of glycolysis, pyruvate, but there are several steps that differ from glycolysis (Figure 3-1). First, instead of the single reaction of **phosphoenolpyruvate (PEP)** donating a phosphate for substrate phosphorylation of ADP to ATP, there are two reactions. The first is to take pyruvate and form oxaloacetate (of TCA fame) by the addition of CO_2, which is catalyzed by pyruvate carboxylase and requires ATP. Next is the decarboxylation and phosphorylation of oxaloacetate to PEP by PEP carboxykinase, which requires a GTP. Two other enzymes are particular to gluconeogenesis (the rest are identical to glycolysis in the reverse direction). Fructose-1,6-bisphosphatase catalyzes the reaction of fructose-1,6-bisphosphate to fructose-6-phosphate and phosphate. Glucose-6-phosphatase (G6Pase) generates glucose from glucose

6-phosphate (G6P), which are the inverse enzymes of PFK and hexokinase, respectively.

Because all the enzymes of gluconeogenesis are identical to glucose except for pyruvate carboxylase, PEP carboxykinase, fructose-1,6-bisphosphatase, and G6Pase, these enzymes are the site of the control for gluconeogenesis. Pyruvate carboxylase is stimulated by acetyl-CoA and both it and PEP carboxykinase are inhibited by ADP. Just as in glycolysis, much of the control is maintained by activating and inhibiting PFK-1; the same is true for gluconeogenesis in which fructose-1,6-bisphosphatase is stimulated by ATP, citrate, glucagon, and epinephrine and inhibited by AMP and fructose-2,6-bisphosphate. The precursors of pyruvate and/or oxaloacetate for gluconeogenesis can come from lactate, amino acids, fatty acids, lactate, fructose, and galactose.

Pyruvate Carboxylase Deficiency A rare cohort of individuals have diminished or absent function of pyruvate carboxylase. Without this initiating enzyme, the amount of precursors to generate glucose is limited. Only the breakdown products of odd-numbered fatty acids, which can enter the TCA cycle and generate oxaloacetate, can be used in gluconeogenesis. This seriously hinders the ability of the liver to respond to glucagon to generate serum glucose as a fuel for the rest of the body. There is an attempt to compensate by storing increased levels of glycogen, but this does not prevent the myriad signs and symptoms of this syndrome.

Individuals affected often present early in life, before their first birthday, with hypoglycemia, progressive delay in achieving milestones, lethargy, hypotonia, optic atrophy, ataxia, and convulsions, and often succumb to death. A possibly milder form can lead to presentation later in life. The syndrome is suspected with the aforementioned signs and symptoms and further by finding elevated lactate, pyruvate, and alanine. Diagnosis can be confirmed by demonstrating an absence in the enzymatic activity of pyruvate carboxylase in tissue from a liver biopsy.

Glycolysis vs. Gluconeogenesis

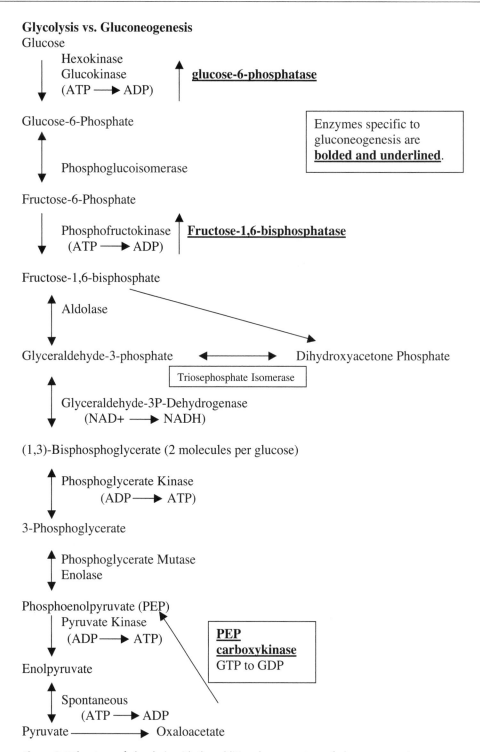

Figure 3-1 The steps of glycolysis with the additional reverse steps of gluconeogenesis.

Case Conclusion   NS is immediately placed on an intravenously (IV) administered D50 to increase her glucose, which in the ED helps her to perk up slightly. A clinical geneticist is consulted and finds that her pyruvate carboxylase activity is minimal. Her parents are advised to feed her often and supplement her diet with thiamine; however, over the ensuing 6 months, she continues to worsen and she dies at age 15 months.

Thumbnail: Gluconeogenesis

Important Reactions in Gluconeogenesis

1. Pyruvate + CO_2 + ATP $\rightarrow$ Oxaloacetate + ADP + P_i (pyruvate carboxylase)
2. Oxaloacetate + GTP $\rightarrow$ PEP + CO_2 + GDP (PEP carboxykinase)
3. Fructose-1,6-diphosphate + H_2O $\rightarrow$ Fructose 6-phosphate + P_i (fructose-1,6-bisphosphatase)
4. G6P + H_2O $\rightarrow$ Glucose + P_i (G6Pase)

Key Points

▶ The four steps in gluconeogenesis that use different enzymes from glycolysis are where the pathway is regulated.

▶ Gluconeogenesis, which occurs in the liver and is stimulated by glucagon and epinephrine, provides glucose for the entire body as glycogen stores are depleted.

▶ A deficiency in the initial enzymes in gluconeogenesis can lead to an excess amount of pyruvate and lactate, causing lactic acidosis in addition to a severe hypoglycemic state.

Questions

1. A patient presents with lethargy, hypotonia, and failure to thrive. An enzymatic assay of hepatic tissue reveals diminished activity of fructose-1,6-bisphosphatase. Which of the following is expected to be decreased?

   A. Fructose-1,6-diphosphate
   B. Glucose
   C. Oxaloacetate
   D. Pyruvate
   E. Acetyl-CoA

2. Without looking back, which of the following enzymes catalyzes a reversible reaction in glycolysis and is used in gluconeogenesis?

   A. Phosphoglucose isomerase
   B. Hexokinase
   C. G6Pase
   D. PK
   E. PFK

3. NS is treated with thiamine for her pyruvate carboxylase deficiency, which of the following might thiamine be expected to help alleviate?

   A. Elevated levels of acetyl-CoA
   B. Metabolic acidosis
   C. Decreased levels of glucose
   D. Hepatomegaly
   E. Deficient myelination

11

HPI: GS is a 9-month-old male infant. He is brought to his primary pediatrician's office for his 9-month checkup. His parents note that although GS eats well and his face and abdomen seem to be growing normally, he does not have the chubby arms and legs that his 11-month-old cousin has.

PE: His head and abdomen are at the fiftieth percentile, but his overall weight and height are below the fifth percentile. He has some yellow plaques on his lower extremities and buttocks. Of note, he has a protuberant abdomen, secondary to an enlarged liver, and consistent with his parents' history, his arms and legs are thin.

Labs: Tests reveal hypoglycemia, with a blood glucose level of 25 mg/dL, increased serum lactate, and both hypertriglyceridemia and hyperuricemia. His CBC count is normal.

Thought Questions

- What are the pathways of glycogen synthesis and degradation?

- How is glycogen used differently in the liver and skeletal muscle?

- What are the different enzyme deficiencies in the various glycogen storage diseases?

Basic Science Review and Discussion

Glycogen is a highly branched molecule composed of glucose molecules linked primarily by α-1,4-glycosidic bonds, but with α-1,6-glycosidic bonds at the branch points. These branch points require a different enzymatic pathway during synthesis and during degradation, which can make glycogen metabolism seem a bit confusing. Essentially, depending on the driving forces in the body, either the storage or the release of glucose is the most important factor.

Glycogen Synthesis   There are two ways for a glucose molecule to be added to a glycogen molecule: either by lengthening a chain by forming an α-1,4-glycosidic linkage or by branching by forming an α-1,6 bond. Before their addition to an enlarging glycogen molecule, a glucose molecule must be energized. This process involves the formation of G6P (by glucokinase in the liver and hexokinase elsewhere). The G6P is converted to glucose 1-phosphate (G1P) by **phosphoglucomutase** and the G1P is converted to **uridine diphosphate glucose** (UDPglucose), catalyzed by **UDPglucose pyrophosphorylase.**

This activated glucose molecule, UDPglucose, can donate a glucose molecule to a glycogen chain with an α-1,4 linkage by the enzyme **glycogen synthase.** A branch point is created after approximately 10 glucose molecules have been added by the enzyme **α-1,4-α-1,6-glucan transferase.** This enzyme breaks an α-1,4 bond and moves the glucose to the α-1,6 site, forming a branch point. Glycogen synthase can then add glucose molecules to this newly formed chain.

Glycogen Degradation   Glycogenolysis requires release of G1P units from the ends of glycogen chains and at the branch points. **Glycogen phosphorylase** catalyzes the phosphorolysis of the α-1,4 bond by addition of a phosphate molecule that releases a G1P molecule. This is the rate-limiting step of glycogen degradation and the principal site of regulation. Once a chain has been broken down to the point where it is approximately four molecules beyond a branch point, **α-1,4-α-1,4-glucan transferase** moves all the glucose molecules from the partially degraded chain except for the branch point molecule to the end of the immediate chain to which it is connected. Then the branch point glucose molecule has its α-1,6-glycosidic bond cleaved by α-1,6-glucosidase. These two enzymes working together are considered the debranching enzymes, or debranching system. The G1P molecule can be converted back to G6P by phosphoglucomutase. The G6P can be used by muscle cells in glycolysis; however, in the liver, the G6P is broken down to glucose plus phosphate by G6Pase. The free glucose can then be transported out of the hepatic cells into the serum.

Regulation of Glycogenesis and Glycogenolysis   Glycogen phosphorylase is activated by phosphorylation of a serine side chain. This activation is precipitated by glucagon in the liver or epinephrine in muscle cells, both leading to increased intracellular cycle AMP (cAMP). Through a cascade mechanism, cAMP-dependent protein kinase A phosphorylates and activates phosphorylase kinase, which in turn phosphorylates glycogen phosphorylase. The active form of glycogen phosphorylase can be allosterically inhibited by ATP and glucose and activated by AMP.

In contrast, glycogen synthase is deactivated by phosphorylation that occurs through a similar pathway to the phosphorylation of glycogen phosphorylase. In this way, the same initiating steps of epinephrine or glucagon leading to activation of protein kinase A result in the opposite effect on these two enzymes. Glycogen synthase can be allosterically activated by G6P.

Glycogen Usage in Different Tissues   Glycogen is primarily stored, synthesized, and catabolized in the liver and skeletal muscle. In the liver, glycogen is used primarily to regulate blood glucose levels. After meals with increased levels of blood glucose, glycogenesis is initiated and the excess glucose is stored in the form of glycogen. As blood glucose levels decrease, glycogenolysis can be initiated and can provide glucose for up to 12 hours. While the liver is maintaining glucose levels for the entire body, glycogen storage in skeletal muscle is used to maintain a local fuel source for the highly metabolic cells. Fast-twitch (white) muscle cells release glucose from glycogen and generate ATP via glycolysis, with the end product being lactic acid. Slow-twitch (red) muscle cells, which are mitochondria rich, use the TCA cycle to generate many-fold more ATP from each glucose molecule.

Glycogen Storage Diseases   There are a number of primary glycogen storage diseases, which each have an enzyme deficiency in either the synthesis or the degradation of glycogen. These diseases can range in presentation from hypoglycemia and muscle cramps to severe hypotonia and infant or early childhood death. The most common disease types and enzyme deficiencies are denoted in Table 4-1.

von Gierke's Disease   GS in the case presentation presents with von Gierke's disease. This is an autosomal recessive (AR) disease resulting in a deficiency of G6Pase. Without G6Pase in the liver, the final step of glycogen breakdown to glucose cannot occur. This leads to increased levels of G6P

Table 4-1

Glycogen storage disease	Enzyme deficiency
Type IA—von Gierke	Glucose-6-phosphatase
Type IB	G6P microsomal translocase
Type II—Pompe	α-1,4-glucosidase
Type III—Cori	Debranching enzyme
Type IV—Andersen	Branching enzyme
Type V—McArdle	Glycogen phosphorylase (muscle)
Type VI—Hers' disease	Glycogen phosphorylase (liver)
Type VII	Phosphofructokinase (muscle)
Type VIII	Phosphorylase kinase (liver)

and G1P and thus increased levels of glycogen stores in the liver. The G6P can enter glycolysis in the liver, and the end product, lactate, enters the serum. The decreased amount of circulating glucose for bioenergetics leads to increased lipid and protein metabolism. Hyperuricemia develops both from decreased renal clearance and from increased production. Long term, these problems can lead to renal failure, growth disturbances, platelet dysfunction, and anemia. Diagnosis is commonly made by liver biopsy, which reveals increased glycogen in the cytoplasm and lipid vacuoles. Type IA disease is confirmed by testing for G6Pase enzyme activity in the biopsy tissue.

Case Conclusion   GS' pediatrician is able to put the constellation of symptoms and laboratory findings together to suspect a glycogen storage disease. He obtains a metabolic consult and a liver biopsy is arranged. This biopsy confirms what is suspected and a diagnosis of von Gierke's disease is made. The primary treatment for this disease is frequent feeding, often continuous tube feeds at night with a mixture of 60% carbohydrates. Cornstarch is commonly used as the primary source of carbohydrates for these patients. GS begins on this dietary regimen provided by his vigilant parents and continues to obtain his developmental milestones over the ensuing year.

Thumbnail: Glycogen Synthesis and Degradation

Important Steps in Glycogen Metabolism

Glycogen synthesis:

Step in pathway	Enzyme
Glucose → G6P	Glucokinase (liver) Hexokinase (muscle)
G6P → G1P	Phosphoglucomutase
G1P + Uridine triphosphate (UTP) → UDPglucose + PPi	UDPglucose pyrophosphorylase
(Glucose)$_n$ + UDPglucose → (Glucose)$_{n+1}$ + UDP	Glycogen synthase
Glycogen chain → Branched chain	α-1,4-α-1,6-glucan transferase

Glycogen degradation:

Step in pathway	Enzyme
(Glucose)$_n$ → (Glucose)$_{n-1}$ + G1P	Glycogen phosphorylase
α-1,4 in branch → α-1,4 linkage in chain	α-1,4-α-1,4-glucan transferase
α-1,6 branch → Glycogen chain + glucose	α-1,6-glucosidase

Key Points

▶ Glycogen metabolism in the liver is used to maintain serum glucose levels.

▶ Glycogen storage in muscle cells provides a ready source of glucose for fiber contractions.

▶ Glycogen metabolism is regulated by activating and deactivating two key enzymes, glycogen phosphorylase and glycogen synthase.

▶ Glycogen storage diseases result from the inability to either store or break down glycogen. The resulting signs and symptoms are dependent on how severe the lack of glucose stores are.

Questions

1. An 11-month-old infant presents to the ED with likely gastroenteritis. Because of vomiting, the parents do not think the infant has kept anything down for 24 hours. Their infant has been extremely lethargic and difficult to arouse. On exam, he has a protuberant abdomen. Laboratory tests reveal hypoglycemia, elevated lactate, hyperuricemia, and hypertriglyceridemia. After he is stabilized for several days, a liver biopsy is performed and his G6Pase activity is normal. His most likely diagnosis is which of the following?

   A. Type IA, von Gierke's disease
   B. Type IB, G6P microsomal translocase deficiency
   C. Type III, Cori's disease
   D. Type VI, Hers' disease
   E. Type V, McArdle's disease

2. A 17-year-old male presents with complaints of severe muscle cramps and weakness after running. He notes that he has had mild cramping after running for several years, but as he increased the distance run over the last few months, he has had increased severity of symptoms. He has attempted to treat the cramps with potassium supplementation to no avail. He is most likely to have which of the following glycogen storage diseases?

   A. Type I, von Gierke's disease
   B. T ype II, Pompe's disease
   C. Type III, Cori's disease
   D. Type IV, Andersen's disease
   E. Type V, McArdle's disease

3. The patient in question 2 is suspected of having one of the glycogen storage diseases. By what intervention will the diagnosis be made?

   A. Liver biopsy and assessing phosphorylase kinase activity
   B. Liver biopsy and assessing glycogen phosphorylase activity
   C. Muscle biopsy and assessing glycogen phosphorylase activity
   D. Genetic testing for mutation on chromosome arm 6
   E. Body CT to measure muscle versus hepatic mass

> **HPI:** LA is a 13-year-old boy who is brought by his mother to an optometrist. He has had rapid deterioration in his vision over the past 2 months. At first, he noticed the vision in his left eye was blurry and his mother noticed him rubbing this eye frequently. After several weeks, the vision in his right eye also became blurry, and he now notices that colors "don't look right."
>
> **PE:** He has noticeable nystagmus. On ophthalmologic exam, he has papilledema and circumpapillary telangiectatic microangiopathy. His optometrist sends him to an ophthalmologist, who among other things orders a serum lactate.

Thought Questions

- Of what diagnoses are the optometrist and ophthalmologist suspicious?

- What are the steps of the electron transport chain (ETC)?

- How does the ETC produce ATP?

- How is this process regulated?

Basic Science Review and Discussion

Leber's hereditary optic neuropathy (LHON) results from mitochondrial mutations that lead to disruptions in complexes I and III of the **ETC.** For example, more than 50% of individuals have a point mutation at nucleotide position 11,778, which leads to a substitution of histidine for arginine in complex I. This leads to a disruption in ATP production and a buildup of NADH. The lack of ATP can lead to damage to the optic nerve and a buildup of lactic acid secondary to inhibition of pyruvate dehydrogenase from NADH buildup. To better understand how LHON can affect bioenergetics, we need to review the ETC and oxidative phosphorylation.

ATP Production from Oxidative Phosphorylation   The ETC converts the NADH and $FADH_2$ produced in glycolysis, the TCA cycle, and oxidation of fatty acids back into their oxidized states. This is done in a sequence of steps, and energy produced by several of these steps is used to produce ATP via oxidative phosphorylation. Although this process is not particularly efficient (only 40% of the energy produced is used to make ATP), without it, ATP production from catabolism is decreased dramatically.

NADH Shuttles   The NADH produced in the cytoplasm needs to be brought into the mitochondria to undergo oxidative phosphorylation. There are two shuttles, the **malate shuttle** and the **α-glycerol phosphate shuttle.** NADH can be oxidized in the production of malate from oxaloacetate, and malate is then shuttled across the mitochondrial membrane. Once inside, malate regenerates both the NADH and the oxaloacetate. The latter is converted to aspartate and shuttled back into the cytosol. The NADH can then enter the ETC. Dihydroxyacetone phosphate conversion to α-glycerol phosphate

also oxidizes NADH, and then α-glycerol phosphate can be shuttled across the mitochondrial membrane. However, once inside, the regeneration of dihydroxyacetone phosphate produces an $FADH_2$ molecule instead of an NADH. This leads to one less ATP per molecule shuttled from the α-glycerol phosphate as compared with the malate shuttle.

Electron Transport Chain   There are four enzyme complexes and two sole enzymes (coenzyme Q [CoQ] and cytochrome c) that compose the ETC. NADH enters the ETC via complex I and in so doing produces one ATP. Succinate enters the ETC via complex II (which is succinate dehydrogenase from TCA cycle fame), which does not produce an ATP. CoQ is the common entry site for NADH after complex I, succinate after complex II (because it produces an $FADH_2$), and $FADH_2$. All three can then go on to complex III, cytochrome c, and complex IV in sequence. This latter process generates two ATP and the reduced oxygen produces H_2O.

ATP Synthase   It has been proposed that ATP is produced via a proton motive force secondary to the proton gradient produced by the ETC. Thus, because complex II does not produce protons, it cannot produce ATP. However, complexes I, III, and IV each produce protons that create a gradient across the inner mitochondrial membrane. ATP synthase, or complex V, couples with this proton gradient at the inner mitochondrial membrane and uses the chemiosmotic energy to produce ATP. ATP synthase is composed of two subunits, a proton channel (F0) and an enzyme that catalyzes ADP to ATP (F1) in the presence of a proton gradient.

Leber's Hereditary Optic Neuropathy   Although LHON was described 100 years ago, the genetic etiology of LHON has just recently been determined. Point mutations in the mitochondrial DNA (mtDNA) lead to either single amino acid substitutions or the disruption of a stop codon, which fundamentally changes the polypeptide produced. This disrupts the enzymes in the ETC, leading to decreased ATP production and buildup of NADH in particular. Exactly how these changes lead to LHON is not entirely clear. Because the mtDNA is in the mitochondria, which are derived solely from the mother (passed from ova to offspring), inheritance is via mitochondrial inheritance. Interestingly, men are affected at a much higher rate than women; essentially 50% of men with the defect will have the disease, and only 20% of women will.

Case Conclusion LA's vision proceeded to worsen over the ensuing 2 years and he developed a large central scotoma. Because of this, he is legally blind and unable to drive. However, he is still able to ambulate and even read with the aid of corrective lenses.

Thumbnail: Oxidative Phosphorylation

NADH and FADH$_2$ in the ETC

NADH

Sources: NADH from TCA, oxidation of fatty acids, malate shuttle from cytosol

NADH $\Rightarrow$ Complex I (ATP) $\Rightarrow$ CoQ $\Rightarrow$ Complex III (ATP) $\Rightarrow$ Complex IV (ATP)

Net production of three ATP molecules per NADH molecule

FADH$_2$

Sources: FADH$_2$ from TCA, fatty acid oxidation, α-glycerol phosphate shuttle from cytosol

FADH$_2$ $\Rightarrow$ CoQ $\Rightarrow$ Complex III (ATP) $\Rightarrow$ Complex IV (ATP)

Net production of two ATP per FADH$_2$ molecule

Key Points

▶ Not all NADH molecules are created equal; for that produced in the cytosol that uses the α-glycerol phosphate shuttle, only three ATP are generated as compared with the malate shuttle.

▶ Oxidative phosphorylation involves the transfer of electrons to oxygen, producing H$_2$O and ATP.

▶ Oxidative phosphorylation is accomplished by a series of enzyme complexes, coenzymes, and cytochromes.

Questions

1. A catabolic process produces two NADH in the cytosol that enter the mitochondria via the α-glycerol phosphate shuttle and a pyruvate that enters the mitochondria and leads to one turn of the TCA cycle. How many ATP molecules will be produced?

   A. 14
   B. 16
   C. 18
   D. 19
   E. 21

2. The mother of LA, the patient from this case, understands that LHON is a genetic disease. She is concerned about the risk to LA's children (her grandchildren). You tell her there is what percentage chance that his children will be affected (assuming his future wife has no mutations)?

   A. 0%
   B. 25%
   C. 33%
   D. 50%
   E. 100%

3. A patient has an enzyme deficiency that leads to a disruption in the α-glycerol phosphate shuttle. In this patient, how many ATP will be produced for each molecule of glucose catabolized?

   A. 2
   B. 6
   C. 12
   D. 22
   E. 32

HPI: FA is a 7-month-old infant who has been increasingly lethargic over the past month. Her anxious parents bring her to the ED because when they went to wake her this morning for her feeding after sleeping for 8 hours straight, she was difficult to awaken. After being awake for several minutes, she had some twitching and jerking of her arms and legs and was even more difficult to awaken over the next 30 minutes. Her parents note that her pregnancy and birth were entirely normal, and that her weight gain has been within normal limits over the past 7 months. They are particularly anxious because their first child died of sudden infant death syndrome (SIDS) at age 9 months.

PE: She is afebrile with normal vital signs. Her head, eyes, ears, nose, throat (HEENT), thoracic, cardiac, and pulmonary exams show no abnormalities. Of note, she has a protuberant abdomen secondary to an enlarged liver.

Labs: Hypoglycemia, with a blood glucose level of 28 mg/dL, metabolic acidosis with increased anion gap, but low ketone bodies. Uric acid is elevated, but her alanine transferase (ALT) and aspartate transferase (AST) levels are normal. Her urine reveals no ketones and increased medium-chain dicarboxylic acids. Her CBC count is normal.

Thought Questions

- What does FA most likely have, and what are the key elements of this disease?

- How are fatty acids synthesized?

- What are the key steps in β-oxidation of fatty acids?

- How are fatty acid synthesis and oxidation controlled?

Basic Science Review and Discussion

Medium-chain acyl-CoA dehydrogenase (MCAD) deficiency is a disease that is caused by an inability to use the fatty acid stores of the body as a fuel source. In particular, because there are short-, medium-, and long-chain fatty acids, MCAD is necessary for C4-to-C14 fatty acid oxidation. Because the long-chain fatty acids need to go through these chain lengths, this diminishes the amount of energy that obtained from storage as medium- or long-chain fatty acids. To better understand the syndrome, we present a brief overview of fatty acid synthesis and oxidation.

Fatty Acids Fatty acids are amphiphilic molecules (both polar and nonpolar) composed of a hydrocarbon chain with a carboxyl group at one terminus. In humans, the important fatty acids generally have an even number of carbons, except propionic acid, which has three. Saturated fatty acids have no double bonds, monounsaturated fatty acids contain one double bond, and polyunsaturated fatty acids contain two or more double bonds. Although many fatty acids can be synthesized, some are considered essential fatty acids, such as linoleic acid (C6=C3=C8 — COOH, where the double bonds are indicated by an equal sign) and can only be obtained from the diet. Fatty acids are primarily stored as triacylglycerols, which are glycerol (C3) backbones with ester linkage to three fatty acids.

Fatty Acid Synthesis The synthesis of fatty acids takes place in the cytosol, but its major fuel, acetyl-CoA, is created inside mitochondria. Because the mitochondrial membrane is impermeable to acetyl-CoA, it is shuttled across with the citrate shuttle. This involves the entrance step of the TCA cycle where citrate is made from acetyl-CoA and oxaloacetate. The citrate molecule then is able to cross the mitochondrial membrane. Once in the cytosol, it can decompose into oxaloacetate and acetyl-CoA. The oxaloacetate further decomposes to pyruvate, which crosses back inside the mitochondria, but the acetyl-CoA molecule can enter into fatty acid synthesis. The first step of this is catalyzed by **acetyl-CoA carboxylase,** which converts acetyl-CoA to **malonyl-CoA** by the addition of a carboxyl group from bicarbonate. Malonyl-CoA then acts to donate two carbon units during the elongation step of fatty acid synthesis. **Fatty acid synthase** acts to catalyze the rest of fatty acid synthesis. It is a multienzyme complex that cycles through four distinct steps in order to donate two carbon units from malonyl-CoA to an elongating fatty acid chain. Acetyl-CoA is bound to the synthase component and added to malonyl-S-acyl carrier protein (ACP) via **condensation to form acetoacetyl-S-ACP.** This then undergoes reduction, dehydration, and a second reduction to become butyryl-S-ACP (butyric acid is a four-carbon fatty acid). The butyryl-CoA can then be transferred to the synthase component and condensed with another malonyl-CoA to elongate the chain. This is generally repeated until the saturated fatty acid palmitoyl-CoA is formed. Palmitoyl-CoA can continue synthesis of longer fatty acids in the endoplasmic reticulum using acetyl-CoA and malonyl-CoA as carbon donors. Unsaturated fats can be synthesized in the endoplasmic reticulum by undergoing desaturation reactions.

Oxidation of Fatty Acids In opposition to synthesis, fatty acid oxidation takes place primarily in the mitochondria. Fatty acids are transported into the mitochondria from the cytosol via the carnitine shuttle. This involves two enzymes and a transporter. Carnitine acyltransferase-I (CAT-I) combines fatty acyl-CoA with carnitine to form fatty acylcarnitine. Carnitine translocase then transports fatty acylcarnitine into the mitochondria. Finally, CAT-II re-forms the activated fatty acyl-CoA in the mitochondria.

Once inside the mitochondria, the fatty acid can undergo β-oxidation of fatty acids, which sequentially removes two carbon fragments from the carboxyl end of the molecule. β-Oxidation involves a cycle of four steps, the net result from each turn of the cycle is an acetyl-CoA, NADH, and $FADH_2$. The steps (illustrated here) are as follows:

$R - C - C - C(=O) - S\text{-CoA}$ (Fatty acyl-CoA) →
$R - C = C - C(=O) - S\text{-CoA}$ (Enoyl-CoA) + $FADH_2$

Dehydrogenation: Formation of a double bond between the α and β carbon generates $FADH_2$.

$R - C = C - C(=O) - S\text{-CoA} + H_2O →$
$R - C(OH) - C - C(=O) - S\text{-CoA}$ (β-hydroxyacyl-CoA)

Hydration: Adds H_2O to the double bond, and OH to the β carbon.

$R - C(OH) - C - C(=O) - S\text{-CoA} →$
$R - C(=O) - C - C(=O) - S\text{-CoA}$ (β-ketoacyl-CoA) + NADH

Dehydrogenation: Converts OH to =O and NADH.

$R - C(=O) - C - C(=O) - S\text{-CoA} + CoASH →$
$R - C(=O) - S\text{-CoA} + C - C(=O) - S\text{-CoA}$ (acetyl-CoA)

Thiolytic cleavage: Adds CoA-SH to the β carbon and releases acetyl-CoA.

The end result of β-oxidation of fatty acids with an odd number of carbons is propionyl-CoA, which can be converted first to methylmalonyl-CoA and then succinyl-CoA, which can enter into the TCA cycle. For a fatty acid with an even number of carbons, $2n$, the net production of acetyl-CoA molecules is n and the number of NADH and $FADH_2$ is $(n - 1)$ each. So for a fatty acid with 16 carbons, 8 acetyl-CoA, 7 NADH, and 7 $FADH_2$ would be produced. Each acetyl-CoA then can enter the TCA cycle and generate 12 ATP. Because the fatty acid requires two ATP to undergo activation, the addition of the high-energy thiol ester bond to Co-ASH, the net production is then $5*(n) + 12*(n-1) - 2$ for a fatty acid with $2n$ carbons.

Regulation of Fatty Acid Metabolism   In fatty acid synthesis, the enzyme that catalyzes the first step, **acetyl-CoA carboxylase**, is the prime point of control. It is activated by citrate, insulin, and increased carbohydrate availability, and it is inhibited by glucagon and increased fatty acid availability. Its synthesis is actually induced by insulin. β-Oxidation of fatty acids is controlled primarily by controlling the flow of fatty acids across the mitochondrial membrane. CAT-I, which is responsible for bringing fatty acids into the mitochondria, is inhibited by malonyl-CoA. Generally, fatty acid oxidation will be decreased by insulin and increased by glucagon.

MCAD Deficiency   The gene for MCAD is located on chromosome I 1p31. Many MCAD gene variants have been reported, but one, the K304E MCAD mutation, accounts for the majority of MCAD mutations identified to date. MCAD is an AR disorder; therefore, individuals who are homozygous or compound heterozygous for an MCAD mutation may have abnormal protein product and subsequent inefficient enzymatic activity to metabolize medium-chain fatty acids. It is estimated that 1 of 80 individuals is a carrier for an MCAD mutation. Whites of northern European descent exhibit the highest frequency of MCAD deficient genotypes.

Clinical Manifestations   MCAD-deficient patients are at risk of the following outcomes: hypoglycemia, vomiting, lethargy, encephalopathy, respiratory arrest, hepatomegaly, seizures, apnea, cardiac arrest, coma, and sudden death. Long-term outcomes may include developmental and behavioral disability, chronic muscle weakness, failure to thrive, cerebral palsy, and attention deficit disorder (ADD). Although there are a number of different gene mutations, the different phenotypic presentations of these mutations have not been determined. Furthermore, the penetrance of MCAD mutations is unclear because there are a number of patients who have the same MCAD deficiency as their siblings without developing the same clinical symptoms in type or severity. Often, a precipitating factor is needed for clinical symptoms to develop; particularly, it is in times of stress, secondary to fasting, increased activity, or illness such as infection, where metabolic demands are higher.

There has been much concern regarding the risk of SIDS in both homozygotes and heterozygotic carriers of the MCAD deficiency mutation, particularly the most common K304E mutation. Recent studies suggest that although there is an increase in the incidence of SIDS in homozygotic patients, there does not seem to be an increase in the prevalence of MCAD mutation carriers among infants with SIDS.

Diagnosis   MCAD mutations can be identified through DNA-based tests using polymerase chain reaction (PCR) and therefore can be detected in patients by DNA analysis. When identification of the K304E mutation is used for diagnostic purposes, detection of homozygosity confirms diagnosis of MCAD deficiency; those heterozygotic for K304E will need confirmation of a second MCAD allelic variant. Mass screening for MCAD deficiency, however, is generally conducted with the detection of abnormal metabolites in urine or blood by tandem mass spectrometry (MS/MS). Typically, MS/MS is used as an initial screening modality followed by confirmation of MCAD deficiency with a urine organic acid profile or DNA mutation analysis.

Treatment and Prognosis Treatment of MCAD deficiency is primarily by both timing and content of diet. In infants and children, whose metabolic demands are higher, it is important for them to have regular meals, generally no more than 6 to 8 hours between them. This issue is more important when they undergo a period of metabolic stress such as an illness. As with other fatty acid deficiencies, supplemen-tation of the diet with carnitine is also instituted. If the disease is identified early before too many hypoglycemic events have caused brain injury, treatment with diet can lead to a much improved prognosis. Others will unfortunately experience developmental delay, behavioral disorders, and cerebral palsy.

Case Conclusion FA is started on frequent feedings, including cornstarch before nighttime sleep and carnitine supple-mentation. Her lethargy improves and she has no further seizure activity. By age 2 years, she is walking, speaking words and short phrases, and appears well.

Thumbnail: Fatty Acid Metabolism

Important Steps in Fatty Acid Metabolism

Fatty acid synthesis

Step in pathway	Enzyme	Bioenergetics
Acetyl-CoA + HCO_3^- → Malonyl-CoA	Acetyl-CoA carboxylase	Requires one ATP
C2n-S-ACP + Malonyl-CoA → C2(n+1)-S-ACP	Fatty acid synthase	Requires two NADPH
Total		
8 acetyl-CoA + HCO_3^- → Palmitoyl-CoA (C16)		Requires 7 ATP + 14 NADPH

Fatty acid oxidation

Step in pathway	Enzyme	Bioenergetics
Activation		
adding CoASH, and using ATP → AMP + PPi → AMP + 2 Pi	Fatty acyl-CoA synthetase	Two ATP equivalents used
Transfer to mitochondria		
Fatty acyl-CoA + Carnitine → Fatty acylcarnitine	CAT-I	None
Fatty acylcarnitine into the mitochondria	Carnitine translocase	None
Fatty acylcarnitine → Fatty acyl-CoA + Carnitine	CAT-II	None
β-Oxidation of fatty acids		
Dehydrogenation forms enoyl-CoA	Fatty acyl-CoA dehydrogenases	$FADH_2$ generated
Hydration forms → β-Hydroxyacyl-CoA		
Dehydrogenation forms β-ketoacyl-CoA		NADH generated
Thiolytic cleavage forms shorter fatty acyl-CoA plus acetyl-CoA		

Key Points

▶ Fatty acids are used both in synthesis of other biologically important molecules and as a source of fuel.

▶ The oxidation of fatty acids yields acetyl-CoA, which can enter the TCA cycle.

▶ MCAD deficiency is the result of a mutation in the fatty acyl-CoA dehydrogenase enzyme responsible for the first step of β-oxidation of fatty acids.

Questions

1. In the setting of MCAD deficiency, one of the aspects of treatment is carnitine diet supplementation, this is important to overcome which of the following?

   A. A total body deficiency of carnitine seen in these patients
   B. A carnitine deficiency in the mitochondria
   C. A carnitine deficiency in the cytosol
   D. The down-regulation of fatty acyl-CoA activity in the cytosol
   E. The decreased acetyl-CoA for the TCA cycle, by entering into TCA at a later step

2. A total of 81% of MCAD-deficient individuals are homozygous for the K304E mutation, 18% are heterozygous for the K304E mutation, and 1% of MCAD-deficient patients do not have the K304E mutation. Given this information, using Hardy-Weinberg formulations, what percentage of MCAD gene mutations are the non-K304E mutation?

   A. 10%
   B. 20%
   C. 30%
   D. 40%
   E. 50%

3. A patient with type I diabetes presents for a visit with her primary care provider. While waiting in her reception area, the patient gives herself an insulin shot and eats her lunch with 45 g of carbohydrates. If her physician sent labs, which of the following would be the correct change secondary to insulin's activity?

   A. Increased fatty acyl-CoA synthetase activity
   B. Decreased CAT-I activity
   C. Increased CAT-II activity
   D. Decreased acetyl-CoA carboxylase synthesis
   E. Increased protein catabolism

HPI: AG is a newborn infant who presents with fused labia majora and clitoromegaly. AG is the product of a normal, full-term pregnancy to a 29-year-old white mother. On day 3 of life while still hospitalized for evaluation of these anomalies, AG becomes listless and exhibits the classic "failure to thrive" syndrome.

PE: AG weighs 3050 g, 350 g less than birth weight, and has a normal blood pressure (BP). While being evaluated for these signs, AG is placed on an IV drip and laboratory tests are sent.

Labs: The immediate lab results reveal low serum sodium and potassium levels, high urinary fractional excretion of sodium (FeNa) level, and elevated serum 17α-hydroxyprogesterone, but decreased 11-deoxycortisol. Serum adrenocorticotropic hormone (ACTH) level and karyotype are pending.

Thought Questions

- What are the pathways of steroid biosynthesis?

- What organs produce steroid hormones?

- What enzyme deficiencies can lead to congenital adrenal hyperplasia (CAH)?

- In CAH, what hormones need to be replaced?

Basic Science Review and Discussion

Steroid biosynthesis occurs in the ovaries, testes, and adrenal cortex. All of the steroid hormones are derived from a single precursor, cholesterol. **Cholesterol** is converted to **pregnenolone** by an enzyme known as either **20,22-desmolase,** or cholesterol side-chain cleavage enzyme. Pregnenolone can then be converted either to **progesterone** or to **17α-hydroxypregnenolone** depending on what pathway the precursor is entering.

Mineralocorticoid Biosynthesis In mineralocorticoid synthesis, pregnenolone is converted to progesterone by **3β-hydroxysteroid dehydrogenase.** This occurs in the adrenal cortex in the outer region known as the zona glomerulosa. The next two steps in this pathway are catalyzed by enzymes common to glucocorticoid synthesis, **21-hydroxylase** and **11β-hydroxylase** (Figure 7-1). The final two steps (which rarely have enzymatic deficiencies) are carried out to produce aldosterone.

Glucocorticoid Biosynthesis Cortisol, the final product from glucocorticoid synthesis, can be produced from either progesterone or 17α-hydroxypregnenolone in the zona fasciculata. **17α-Hydroxylase** can catalyze the production of 17α-hydroxypregnenolone from pregnenolone or 17α-hydroxyprogesterone from progesterone. 17α-Hydroxyprogesterone can also be produced from 17α-hydroxypregnenolone by 3β-hydroxysteroid dehydrogenase. 21-Hydroxylase and 11β-hydroxylase then convert 17α-hydroxyprogesterone to **cortisol.**

Sex Hormone Biosynthesis Sex hormones are synthesized in the adrenal cortex in the zona reticularis or in the ovaries or testes. The enzyme **17,20-desmolase** can convert either 17α-hydroxypregnenolone or 17α-hydroxyprogesterone to androgenic precursors. The androgenic hormones testosterone and androstenedione can be converted to estrone and estradiol, respectively, by aromatase. However, aromatase is present only in the ovaries.

Congenital Adrenal Hyperplasia As can be seen in the steroid biosynthetic pathways, if there is a lack of one of the enzymes that lead pregnenolone toward mineralocorticoid or glucocorticoid synthesis, the precursors can be converted to androgens. In women, a small amount of these androgens will be converted to estrogens, but the great majority end up in the peripheral circulation. This leads to the phenotypic findings of virilization seen in this case. In addition, the lack of glucocorticoids and mineralocorticoids can have a disastrous effect, essentially an Addisonian crisis at several days of life. The severity of these findings is associated with the particular enzyme deficiency.

The most common enzyme deficiency leading to **CAH** is that of 21α-hydroxylase. Patients will have symptoms similar to those of AG, and about half will be salt wasting, as AG is. The diagnosis can be confirmed by the elevation of 17α-hydroxyprogesterone without an elevation in 11-deoxycortisol. If the deficient enzyme is 11β-hydroxylase, then 11-deoxycortisol will be elevated.

Patients with CAH need treatment both to replace their missing hormones and to guard against the effects of the excess androgens. Replacement is most commonly with hydrocortisone or prednisone, and patients with salt wasting will also need a mineralocorticoid such as flucortisone. The steroid replacement then acts to both replace missing hormones and produce a negative feedback on ACTH production, diminishing the amount of excess androgens. Females with virilization may require surgical therapy, but often mild effects may reverse with medical therapy.

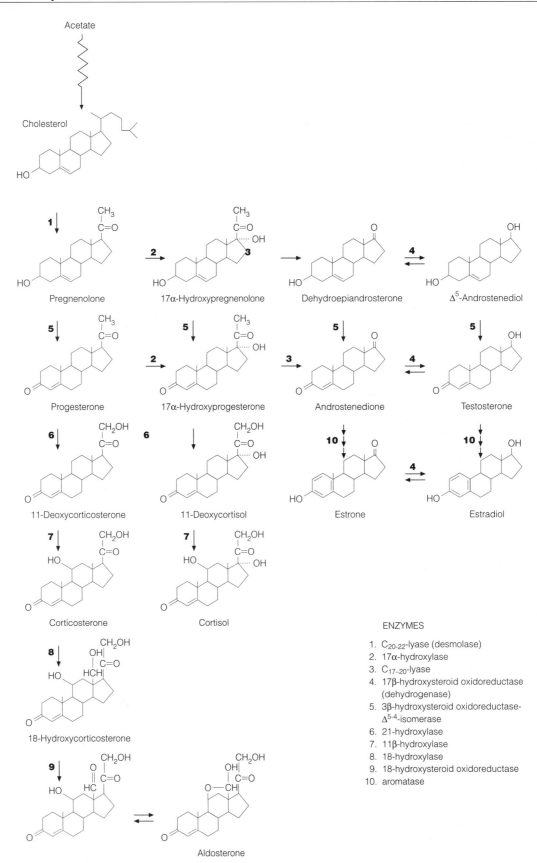

Figure 7-1 The steps in the biosynthesis of the steroid hormones using three primary pathways to generate glucocorticoids, mineralocorticoids, and the sex steroids. (Reproduced with permission from Mishell DR, et al. Infertility, Contraception, and Reproductive Endocrinology. 3rd ed. Malden: Blackwell Science, 1991.)

Case Conclusion AG's karyotype comes back as 46,XX, which reassures her parents that she is indeed a baby girl. Her ACTH level is quite elevated, as are her androstenedione levels. She is given both hydrocortisone and flucortisone, and these levels diminish over the next few weeks. An estrogen cream is placed topically on her labia, and over the next few months, the thin adhesions keeping the labia together resolve, as does her clitoromegaly.

Thumbnail: Steroid Biosynthesis

Important Steps in Steroid Synthesis			
Enzyme	**Pathway**	**Precursor**	**Product**
20,22-Desmolase	Common	Cholesterol	Pregnenolone
21-Hydroxylase	Mineralocorticoid Glucocorticoid	Progesterone 17α-Hydroxyprogesterone	11-Deoxycortisone 11-Deoxycortisol
11β-Hydroxylase	Mineralocorticoid Glucocorticoid	11-Deoxycorticosterone 11-Deoxycortisol	Corticosterone Cortisol
17α-Hydroxylase	Glucocorticoid Sex hormone	Pregnenolone Progesterone	17α-hydroxyprogesterone 17α-hydroxypregnenolone
17,20-Desmolase	Sex hormone	17α-Hydroxypregnenolone 17α-Hydroxyprogesterone	Dehydroepiandrosterone Androstenedione

Key Points

▶ Cholesterol is the common precursor of all the steroid hormones.

▶ A missing enzyme in these biosynthetic pathways leads to both an absence of one hormone and an excess of another.

▶ The most common enzyme deficiency leading to CAH is 21α-hydroxylase.

Questions

1. A 10-day-old boy is diagnosed with a variant of CAH. He is missing the activity of the 11β-hydroxylase enzyme. Which of the following will be elevated?

   A. Cholesterol, pregnenolone, 11-deoxycorticosterone
   B. Cholesterol, pregnenolone, 11-deoxycortisol
   C. Pregnenolone, 11-deoxycortisol, 11-deoxycorticosterone
   D. 11-Deoxycortisol, 11-deoxycorticosterone, estrone
   E. 11-Deoxycortisol, 11-deoxycorticosterone, androstenedione

2. When considering the classic presenting signs, symptoms, and lab abnormalities of CAH, which of the following enzyme deficiencies is likely to cause CAH?

   A. 20,22-Desmolase
   B. 17,20-Desmolase
   C. 3β-Hydroxysteroid dehydrogenase
   D. 18-Hydroxylase
   E. 18-Hydroxysteroid dehydrogenase

HPI: CS is 1-month-old female infant who was born with several congenital anomalies. These include an extra finger on each hand, a cleft lip and palate, and Hirschsprung's disease. Over the past month, she has seen several plastic surgeons regarding repair of these congenital anomalies, and now she is being seen by a genetic specialist because her primary pediatrician is concerned that in addition to these congenital anomalies, she is not feeding well or gaining weight.

PE: The geneticist notes the aforementioned anomalies, in addition to low-set ears, drooping eyelids, and a small upturned nose.

Labs: Concerned for a genetic abnormality, she orders a test for a 7-dehydrocholesterol (7DHC) level, among other tests.

Thought Questions

■ What diagnosis is the geneticist concerned about?

■ How will the 7DHC level help in diagnosis?

■ What are the key steps on the pathway of biosynthesis of cholesterol?

Basic Science Review and Discussion

One of the leading diagnoses with this constellation of findings is **Smith-Lemli-Opitz (SLO) syndrome**. This syndrome is based on a genetic defect in the synthesis of cholesterol; thus, we begin with a review of cholesterol biosynthesis.

Cholesterol Synthesis   The key first steps in **cholesterol synthesis** include two acetyl-CoA molecules combining to make **acetoacetyl-CoA,** which further combines with a third acetyl-CoA to make **hydroxymethylglutaryl-CoA (HMG-CoA)** (Figure 8-1).

A step that is both highly regulated and a primary target for cholesterol-lowering agents is catalyzed by HMG-CoA reductase, which reduces HMG-CoA to **mevalonate** (Figure 8-2). HMG-CoA reductase inhibitors are first-line agents in cholesterol reduction.

Three ATP are then required to take mevalonate to **isopentenylpyrophosphate** in three steps. Isopentenylpyrophosphate is the first of several compounds in the pathway that are referred to as isoprenoids. Isopentenylpyrophosphate isomerase interconverts isopentenylpyrophosphate and dimethylallylpyrophosphate. **Prenyl transferase** catalyzes head-to-tail condensations of dimethylallylpyrophosphate with isopentenylpyrophosphate several times to form farnesyl pyrophosphate. Squalene synthase then performs head-to-head condensation of two farnesyl pyrophosphate molecules to form **squalene** (Figure 8-3). Squalene epoxidase catalyzes oxidation of squalene to form 2,3-oxidosqualene, requiring NADPH as a reductant. Squalene oxidocyclase catalyzes a series of cyclization reactions, producing the sterol **lanosterol** (see Figure 8-3).

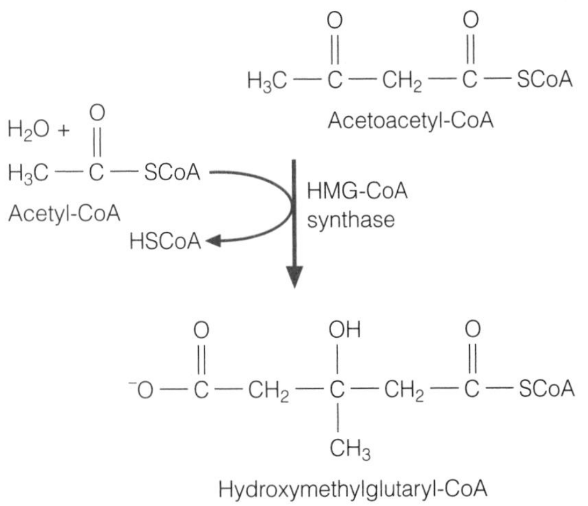

Figure 8-1 Key regulation step in cholesterol synthesis.

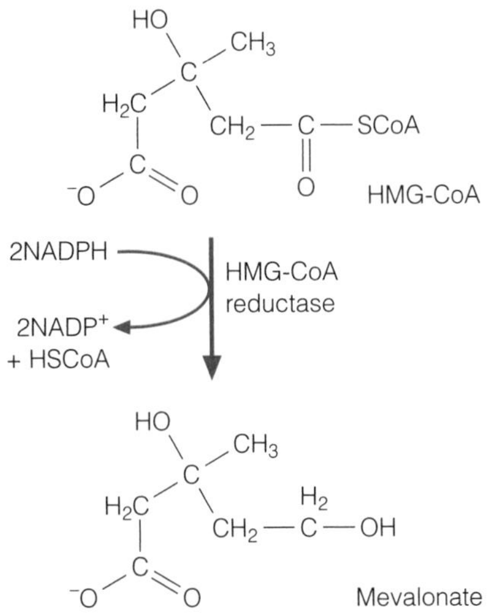

Figure 8-2 Key pharmacologic target, action of HMG-CoA reductase.

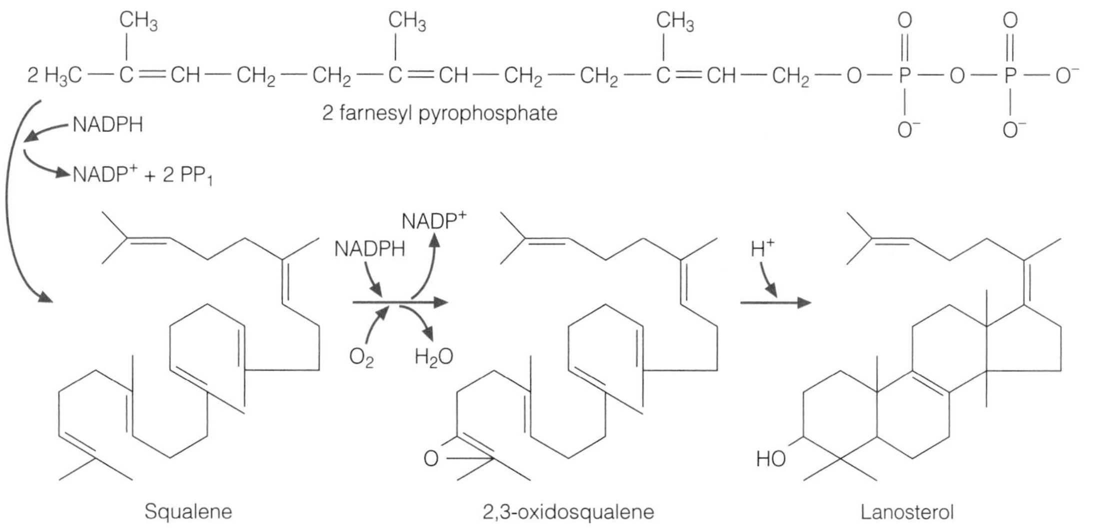

Figure 8-3 Conversion of chain to sterol rings.

The conversion of lanosterol to cholesterol then requires 19 steps. The final step is the conversion of 7DHC to cholesterol. This is catalyzed by **7-dehydrocholesterol-δ-7-reductase (DHCR7).** A defect in this gene is the etiology of SLO syndrome.

Clinical Correlation   SLO syndrome is a genetic disorder that was first described in 1964 in three boys with poor growth, developmental delay, and a common pattern of congenital malformations including cleft palate, genital malformations, and polydactyly (extra fingers and toes). It was not until 1993 that SLO syndrome was determined to be an AR genetic condition caused by deficiency of the enzyme 7-dehydrocholesterol-δ-7-reductase (also known as 3β-hydroxysterol-δ-7-reductase) the final enzyme in the sterol synthetic pathway that converts *7DHC* to cholesterol. This defect in cholesterol production results in a wide set of congenital anomalies, as well as developmental delay. The incidence of SLO syndrome may be as high as 1 of 10,000 to 1 of 20,000 births, with a carrier frequency between 1 of 50 and 1 of 70 individuals.

Currently, the reason defects in cholesterol synthesis cause congenital malformations is not understood. Several disparate lines of research have led to our recent understanding of the critical and somewhat unexpected role of cholesterol in early human development. Cholesterol is important in cell membranes, serves as the precursor for steroid hormones and bile acids, and is a major component in myelin. Cholesterol is covalently bound to the embryonic signaling protein **Sonic hedgehog** (Shh) in a necessary step of the autoprocessing of the precursor to the active form, occurring at about day 0 to 7 estimated gestational age in humans.

Shh plays a critical role in several embryologic fields relevant to SLO syndrome (e.g., brain, face, heart, and limbs).

Therefore, cholesterol is an essential triggering agent in the early developmental program of the human. Because 7DHC also can activate Shh, cholesterol deficiency leading to decreased activation of Shh probably is not the sole explanation for congenital malformations in this syndrome. Abnormalities in the Shh-patched signaling cascade presumably play a role. Membrane instability and dysmyelination from cholesterol deficiency and accumulation of 7DHC and other potentially toxic cholesterol precursors may also contribute to the SLO phenotype.

Diagnosis and Treatment   SLO syndrome is most commonly diagnosed postnatally, but certain congenital anomalies that can be seen on ultrasound (US) may lead a diagnosis to be suspected prenatally. These include polydactyly, cleft palate, hypospadias, cataracts, cardiac anomalies, pyloric stenosis, and microcephaly. Many of these anomalies are missed on a routine US, but others, including low-set ears, abnormal palmar creases, micrognathia, foreshortened thumbs and Hirschsprung's disease, will be missed even on level II US exams. In addition, these anomalies can be seen in other syndromes, thereby making a specific diagnosis quite difficult. Postnatally, the diagnosis becomes easier in the setting of one or more of these anomalies, a 7DHC level can be seen to be elevated. SLO syndrome is increasingly screened for using levels of 7DHC in cultured cells. In addition, a genetic test for the gene defect is being developed and should become available soon. At this point, some states (California) are offering screening to everyone, but others offer it only to anyone with relatives with the syndrome.

Because the problem with SLO syndrome is not just the congenital anomalies, but also an ongoing problem with cholesterol synthesis, there is hope that treatment can be accomplished with dietary cholesterol supplementation. As a result, many children and adults with SLO syndrome are being given supplementary cholesterol, either in a natural form, such as egg yolks and cream, or in the form of purified cholesterol given as part of several research protocols.

Because the accumulation of 7DHC may contribute to some of the effects of SLO syndrome, HMG-CoA reductase inhibitors are beginning to be used to decrease its production in clinical trials, along with cholesterol supplementation. At this point, curative treatments such as gene therapy are purely theoretical.

Case Conclusion CS' lab results reveal an elevated 7DHC level. She is diagnosed with SLO syndrome and her parents are educated about what this diagnosis means for their daughter and future pregnancies. She begins cholesterol supplementation, and the geneticist and the parents begin to look for a clinical trial using HMG-CoA reductase inhibitors to enroll CS.

Thumbnail: Cholesterol Synthesis

Important Steps in the Synthetic Pathway

Acetyl-CoA + acetyl-CoA → Acetoacetyl-CoA

Acetoacetyl-CoA + Acetyl-CoA → HMG-CoA

HMG-CoA → Mevalonate (catalyzed by HMG-CoA reductase)

Mevalonate →→→ Isopentenylpyrophosphate (requires three ATP)

Isopentenylpyrophosphate → dimethylallylpyrophosphate (isopentenylpyrophosphate isomerase)

Isopentenylpyrophosphate and dimethylallylpyrophosphate → Farnesyl pyrophosphate

Farnesyl pyrophosphate + Farnesyl pyrophosphate → Squalene

Squalene → 2,3-Oxidosqualene (squalene epoxidase requires NADPH)

2,3-Oxidosqualene →→ Lanosterol (squalene oxidocyclase in a series of cyclization steps)

Lanosterol → 18 steps → 7-Dehydrocholesterol

7-Dehydrocholesterol → Cholesterol (7-Dehydrocholesterol-δ-7-reductase)

Key Points

▶ The key regulation step in cholesterol synthesis is catalyzed by HMG-CoA reductase.

▶ This step is also a key pharmacologic site for cholesterol-lowering agents.

▶ Cholesterol synthesis requires three ATP molecules and an NADPH molecule for each molecule synthesized.

▶ SLO syndrome results from a defect in 7-dehydrocholesterol-δ-7-reductase, which catalyzes the final step in cholesterol synthesis.

Questions

1. Compared with patients with SLO syndrome, patients on enormously high quantities of HMG-CoA reductase inhibitors would have which of the following?

   A. Lower levels of 7DHC
   B. The same amount of 7DHC
   C. Greater levels of 7DHC
   D. Greater levels of mevalonate
   E. Lower levels of HMG-CoA

2. Without reviewing the steps in the thumbnail, the key regulatory step in cholesterol synthesis is which of the following?

   A. Acetyl-CoA to acetoacetyl-CoA
   B. Acetoacetyl-CoA to HMG-CoA
   C. HMG-CoA to mevalonate
   D. Mevalonate to isopentenylpyrophosphate
   E. 7DHC to cholesterol

> **HPI:** CP is a 29-year-old white man who presents to the ED with chest pain that radiates down his left arm and tingling in his jaw. The symptoms have come and gone at times of stress and exercise for the past year, but the current episode is far worse. His family history includes a deceased maternal grandfather of a heart attack at age 43, as well as a maternal uncle who died of a heart attack at age 38.
>
> **PE:** Chest and abdominal exams show no abnormalities. Inspection of his ankles reveals nodular swellings on his Achilles tendon. An ECG shows evidence of an acute inferior myocardial infarction (IMI).
>
> **Labs:** Results are pending.

Thought Questions

- What genetic diagnoses should the ED doctor consider?

- What key findings help make this diagnosis?

- What are the key elements of lipid digestion, absorption, and transport?

- What is the enterohepatic cycle?

Basic Science Review and Discussion

In patients who do indeed have a myocardial infarction (MI) before the age of 40, **hypercholesterolemia** and **hyperlipidemia** should always be considered in the differential diagnosis. Further strengthening the diagnosis in this patient are the likely **xanthomas** on his tendons, which is seen classically in familial hypercholesterolemia. Before the clinical discussion of these diseases, a brief review of lipid digestion, metabolism, and transport is presented.

Lipid Digestion and Absorption Because most of the body is an aqueous solution, lipids provide a challenge to digestion, absorption, and transport because of their **hydrophobic** nature. The first step of digestion of lipids is enhanced by bile acids secreted by the liver and stored in the gallbladder (Figure 9-1). Bile acids are derivatives of cholesterol with polar components, making them **amphipathic**. This property allows them to solubilize fats and be carried through aqueous solutions. Thus, they are able to emulsify fatty molecules in the gut, providing enzymes better access to them.

One such enzyme is **pancreatic lipase,** which catalyzes hydrolysis of triacylglycerols at their 1 and 3 positions (Figure 9-2), forming 1,2-diacylglycerols and then 2-monoacylglycerols (monoglycerides). Monoacylglycerols and fatty acids are absorbed by intestinal epithelial cells. Within intestinal epithelial cells, triacylglycerols are resynthesized. **Phospholipase A_2** is secreted by the pancreas into the intestine. It hydrolyzes the ester linkage between the fatty acid and the hydroxyl on C2 of phospholipids produc-

ing **lysophospholipids.** These lysophospholipids then aid digestion of other lipids by breaking up fat globules into small micelles.

Enterohepatic Cycle Cholesterol can be readily synthesized and absorbed, but the only way it is metabolized and excreted is via conversion to **bile salts.** These are then secreted into the intestine and used to emulsify and digest fats, and they are most commonly reabsorbed. This process of the secretion, reabsorption, and return to the liver of bile acids is known as the enterohepatic cycle. Evolutionarily, this is important because there was very little dietary cholesterol available to our ancestors, but it provides a source of major morbidity and mortality, with hypercholesterolemia being a risk factor for atherosclerosis and coronary artery disease (CAD). Thus, the interruption of this cycle, which allows cholesterol products to be excreted into the GI tract without reabsorption, may help lower cholesterol. These agents include synthetic resins and soluble fibers.

Lipid Transport Once absorbed by the intestinal cells, cholesterol may be esterified to fatty acids forming cholesteryl esters. This is catalyzed by **acyl-CoA:cholesterol acyltransferase** (ACAT). Fatty acids (which are poorly soluble and have detergent properties) are not bound to cholesterol

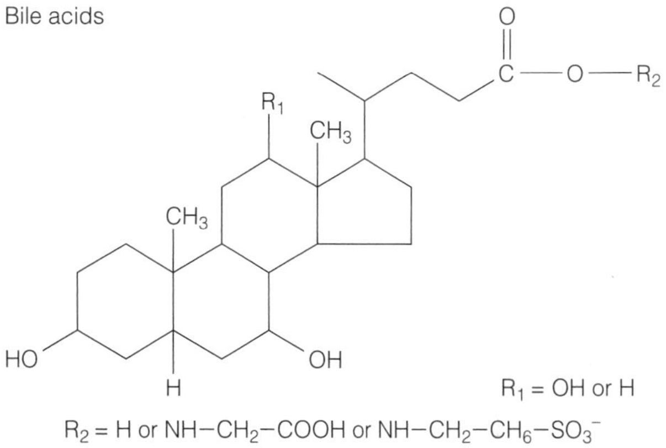

Figure 9-1 Bile acids are amphipathic with both hydrophilic and hydrophobic regions.

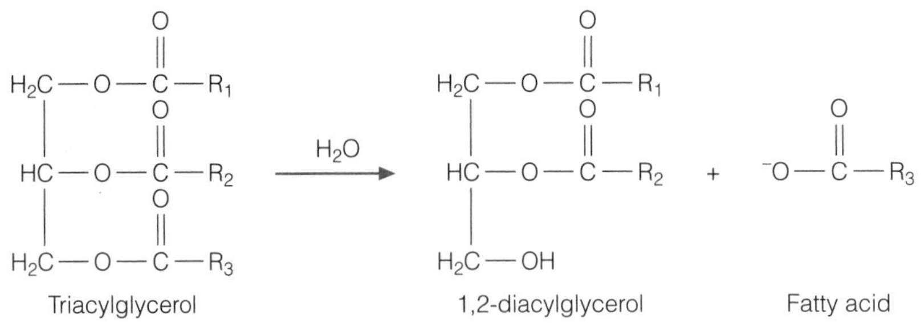

$$H_2C-O-\overset{\overset{\displaystyle O}{\|}}{C}-R_1$$
$$HC-O-\overset{\overset{\displaystyle O}{\|}}{C}-R_2 \xrightarrow{H_2O} HC-O-\overset{\overset{\displaystyle O}{\|}}{C}-R_2 \quad + \quad {}^-O-\overset{\overset{\displaystyle O}{\|}}{C}-R_3$$
$$H_2C-O-\overset{\overset{\displaystyle O}{\|}}{C}-R_3 \qquad H_2C-OH$$

Triacylglycerol　　　　　　1,2-diacylglycerol　　　　Fatty acid

Figure 9-2 Hydrolysis of triacylglycerol.

and thus are kept sequestered from the cytosol by being bound by **intestinal fatty acid-binding protein** (I-FABP) or are transported in the blood bound to **albumin**. Other lipids are transported in the blood as part of **lipoproteins** (Figure 9-3), complex particles whose structure includes a core consisting of a droplet of triacylglycerols and/or cholesteryl esters, as well as a surface monolayer of phospholipid, cholesterol, and specific proteins (apolipoproteins).

Lipoproteins differ in their contents of proteins and lipids. They are classified based on density.

- **Chylomicron:** largest; lowest in density due to high lipid-protein ratio; highest in triacylglycerols as percentage of weight
- **Very-low-density lipoprotein (VLDL):** second highest in triacylglycerols as percentage of weight
- **Intermediate-density lipoprotein (IDL)**
- **Low-density lipoprotein (LDL):** highest in cholesteryl esters as percentage of weight
- **High-density lipoprotein (HDL):** highest in density because of high protein-lipid ratio

After absorbing or synthesizing triacylglycerols, cholesteryl esters, phospholipids, free cholesterol, and apolipoproteins, the epithelial cells lining the intestine package these lipids into **chylomicrons**. The chylomicrons are then secreted and transported via the lymphatic system to the blood.

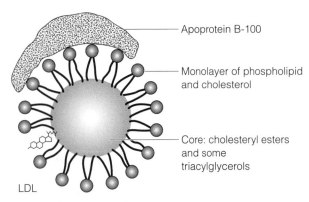

　　　　　　　　　— Apoprotein B-100

　　　　　　　　　— Monolayer of phospholipid
　　　　　　　　　and cholesterol

　　　　　　　　　— Core: cholesteryl esters
　　　　　　　　　and some
　　　　　　　　　triacylglycerols

LDL

Figure 9-3 The structure of LDLs.

Apolipoprotein C-II (apo C-II) on the chylomicron surface activates **lipoprotein lipase,** an enzyme attached to the luminal surface of small blood vessels. Lipoprotein lipase catalyzes hydrolytic cleavage of fatty acids from triacyl glycerols of chylomicrons, and these fatty acids and monoacylglycerols are picked up by body cells for use as energy sources. As triacylglycerols are cleaved and removed through this process, the chylomicrons shrink, becoming **chylomicron remnants** with lipid cores having a relatively high concentration of cholesteryl esters. These chylomicron remnants are taken up by liver cells, via receptor-mediated endocytosis involving recognition of **apo E** of the chylomicron remnant by receptors on the liver cells.

Liver cells produce and secrete into the blood VLDL. The core of this lipoprotein has a relatively high triacylglycerol content. One of the apolipoproteins of VLDL is B-100. Microsomal triglyceride transfer protein (MTP), in the lumen of the endoplasmic reticulum in liver, has an essential role in VLDL assembly. MTP facilitates transfer of lipids to apo B-100 while apo B-100 is being translocated into the endoplasmic reticulum lumen during translation. VLDL assembly is dependent on availability of lipids and apo B-100. As VLDL particles are transported in the bloodstream, **lipoprotein lipase** catalyzes triacylglycerol removal by hydrolysis. With this removal, the percentage weight of cholesteryl esters increases. VLDLs are converted to IDLs, and eventually to LDLs. The lipid core of LDL is predominantly cholesteryl esters. Whereas VLDL contains five apolipoprotein types (apo B-100, apo C-I, apo C-II, apo C-III, and apo E), only one protein, apo B-100, is associated with the surface monolayer of LDL. Cell membranes contain an LDL receptor that binds LDL and leads to endocytosis and absorption of the LDL molecule.

HDL (the cholesterol that is "good" for you) is secreted as a small protein-rich particle by the liver (and intestine). One HDL apolipoprotein, apo A-I, activates **lecithin-cholesterol acyltransferase (LCAT),** which catalyzes synthesis of cholesteryl esters using fatty acids cleaved from the membrane lipid lecithin. The cholesterol is scavenged from cell surfaces & from other lipoproteins. HDL may transfer some cholesteryl esters to other lipoproteins. Some remain associated with HDL, which may be taken up by the liver and degraded. HDL thus transports cholesterol from tissues and other lipoproteins to the liver, which can excrete excess cholesterol as bile acids.

Clinical Correlation A number of enzyme, receptor, and molecular deficiencies can result in syndromes that cause premature atherosclerosis. These include familial hypercholesterolemia, lipoprotein lipase deficiency, hypertriglyceridemia, and hyperlipoproteinemia. The pathophysiology of these are each interesting and depend on the pathways elucidated earlier. Patients with familial hypercholesterolemia, an autosomal dominant (AD) disease that occurs in 1 in 500 individuals, have a mutation in the LDL receptor gene. This leads to elevations in LDL and total cholesterol, because LDL is not bound and endocytosed by cells.

Lipoprotein lipase deficiency (AR) results in diminished metabolism of the chylomicrons and their buildup in the plasma. In patients with type III hyperlipoproteinemia (familial dysbetalipoproteinemia), which is essentially AD, the uptake of IDL and chylomicron remnants is diminished or absent, leading to elevated plasma levels of these lipoproteins. Familial hypertriglyceridemia is also an AD disease in which patients have difficulty in catabolizing VLDL triglycerides. This can lead to elevated triglycerides over time.

Diagnosis and Treatment All of these syndromes result in elevated lipoproteins and/or triglycerides. The two most common clinical presentations are xanthomas and premature **atherosclerosis.** Xanthomas are fatty deposits that are yellow and can erupt anywhere on the body, and certain cases of these syndromes show a clearer pattern of presentation than others. The premature atherosclerosis is most aggressive in familial hypercholesterolemia often presenting in patients in their 20s and 30s as an MI. Still other patients, those with familial apo C-II deficiency will present in childhood with pancreatitis. Patients with family histories of these outcomes should be screened with annual lipid profiles and physical exams, and they should be advised to avoid a high-fat, high-carbohydrate diet, because patients with diabetes and obesity are more likely to experience the complications of this disease.

Although xanthomas can be surgically removed, removal of atherosclerotic plaques in the arteries throughout the body can be more difficult. CAD can be treated as it usually is. The prevention and treatment of these rare diseases can include the use of binding agents (e.g., cholestyramine) to reduce cholesterol and triglyceride absorption and distribution. In the syndromes in which there is primarily a cholesterol elevation, HMG-CoA reductase inhibitors, which block the synthesis of cholesterol at its rate-limiting step, can be used.

Case Conclusion The ED physician, concerned about an acute MI, begins treatment for CP with an aspirin and a beta-blocker to control his BP, and CP is given morphine for his pain. His labs return with an elevated cardiac troponin I and myocardial muscle creatine kinase isoenzyme (CK-MB) elevation, which are both consistent with an acute MI. His triglycerides and LDLs are extremely elevated as well, leading most likely to a diagnosis of familial hypercholesterolemia. The ED physician calls the cardiology fellow to take CP for a cardiac catheterization.

Thumbnail: Cholesterol and Lipid Metabolism

Familial Hyperlipoproteinemias			
Disorder	**Defect**	**Lab elevation**	**Presentation**
Familial hypercholesterolemia	Absent LDL receptor	LDL	Xanthomas on tendons, atherosclerosis
Familial hypertriglyceridemia	?	VLDL	Eruptive xanthomas, atherosclerosis
Familial lipoprotein lipase deficiency	Lipoprotein lipase deficiency	Chylomicrons	Eruptive xanthomas, pancreatitis
Familial type III hyperlipoproteinemia	Abnormal VLDL apo E	Chylomicrons, IDL	Palmar xanthomas, atherosclerosis
Familial apo C-II deficiency	Apo C-II deficiency	Chylomicrons, VLDL	Pancreatitis
Familial combined hyperlipidemia	?	LDL, VLDL	Xanthomas, atherosclerosis

Key Points

▶ Lipid digestion is begun by bile acids which emulsify fatty molecules.

▶ Then enzymes such as pancreatic lipase catalyze hydrolysis of triacylglycerols.

▶ Monoacylglycerols and fatty acids are absorbed by intestinal epithelial cells, and within intestinal epithelial cells, triacylglycerols are resynthesized.

▶ Once absorbed by the intestinal cells, cholesterol may be esterified to fatty acids, forming cholesteryl esters catalyzed by ACAT.

▶ Triacylglycerols, cholesteryl esters, phospholipids, and free cholesterol are packaged into chylomicrons in the GI tract epithelium for transport.

▶ Chylomicrons have these fatty molecules removed by cells throughout the body until they become chylomicron remnants and are absorbed by the liver.

▶ Cholesterol is further transported by VLDL, IDL, LDL, and HDL.

Questions

1. The key step catalyzed by lipoprotein lipase is which of the following?

   A. Hydrolysis of triacylglycerols
   B. Hydrolysis primarily of monoacylglycerols
   C. Conversion of chylomicrons to HDLs
   D. Chylomicron conversion to triacylglycerols
   E. Binding to apo B-100

2. Which of the following patients is most likely to have atherosclerosis, xanthomas, and pancreatitis, but LDL and VLDL levels normal or only slightly elevated?

   A. 65-year-old man who is morbidly obese
   B. 42-year-old man with lipoprotein lipase deficiency
   C. 33-year-old woman with familial hypercholesterolemia
   D. 48-year-old man with familial hypertriglyceridemia
   E. 55-year-old man who smokes and has a family history of heart disease

> **HPI:** JG is a 24-year-old woman who is gravida 1 para 0 at 37 weeks of gestation who presents for a routine prenatal visit. Her pregnancy has been thus far uncomplicated and she has no significant medical problems. She complains of a persistent headache for 2 days, not relieved by acetaminophen (Tylenol). In addition, she complains of "puffiness" of her face and hands. Upon further questioning, she also reveals a 1-day history of right upper quadrant (RUQ) pain.
>
> **PE:** Significant for an elevated BP of 165/92 mm Hg, generalized edema of the face and hands, mild RUQ tenderness, and 3+ reflexes bilaterally.
>
> **Labs:** Office urine dip is notable for 2+ proteinuria.

Thought Questions

- What are the pathways and products of arachidonic acid (AA) metabolism?

- How do the products of AA metabolism affect blood vessels?

- What are potential target areas of AA metabolism for therapy?

Basic Science Review and Discussion

The products of *AA* metabolism are the **eicosanoids,** which include **prostaglandins, thromboxanes (TXA$_2$),** and **leukotrienes.** Eicosanoids are 20-carbon fatty acids that act as local hormones that participate in inflammation and hemostasis following infection or injury. This inflammatory response can produce symptoms including pain, swelling, and fever. Allergic and hypersensitivity reactions represent an exaggerated expression of the normal eicosanoid-mediated inflammatory response.

Functions of Arachidonic Acid Metabolites

- **Smooth muscle contraction:** BP regulation, vasoconstriction **(thromboxane),** bronchial constriction, and uterine contraction.

- **Platelet aggregation: Thromboxane** is a potent enhancer of platelet aggregation. **Prostacyclin** is a potent inhibitor of platelet aggregation.

- **The inflammatory response: Leukotrienes** act as chemotaxic agents, attracting leukocytes to the site of inflammation (Table 10-1). Certain **prostaglandins** mediate pain, fever, sleep, and wakefulness.

Table 10-1 Inflammatory Actions of Eicosanoids

Action	Metabolite
Vasoconstriction	TXA$_2$, LTC$_4$, LTD$_4$, LTE$_4$
Vasodilation	PGI$_2$, PGE$_1$, PGE$_2$, PGD$_2$
Increased vascular permeability	LTC$_4$, D$_4$, E$_4$
Chemotaxis, leukocyte adhesion	LTB$_4$, HETE, lipoxins

Arachidonic Acid Structure and Synthesis AA is a 20-carbon polyunsaturated fatty acid derived from dietary sources or by conversion of **linoleic acid** (an essential fatty acid). It is esterified in membrane phospholipids and released after the activation of cellular **phospholipases** by specific stimuli. AA metabolism proceeds by one of two major pathways named after the enzymes that initiate the reactions: the **cyclooxygenase (COX) pathway** and the **lipoxygenase pathway** (Figure 10-1).

The Cyclooxygenase Pathway The COX pathway, mediated by two enzymes (COX-1 and COX-2), leads to the generation of **prostaglandins.** These include PGE$_2$, PGD$_2$, PGF$_{2\alpha}$, PGI$_2$ (prostacyclin), and TXA$_2$. *PGI$_2$* and *TXA$_2$* have opposing roles. PGI$_2$ is generated by the vascular endothelium and acts as a vasodilator and potent inhibitor of platelet aggregation. TXA$_2$ is produced by platelets and acts as a vasoconstrictor and potent platelet-aggregating factor. PGE$_2$, PGD$_2$, and PGF$_{2\alpha}$ cause vasodilation and potentiate edema formation.

Aspirin and NSAIDs, such as indomethacin and ibuprofen inhibitors, inhibit COX and therefore inhibit prostaglandin synthesis. Glucocorticoids are powerful anti-inflammatory agents that act to inhibit the release of AA from membrane phospholipids. Glucocorticoids affect both the COX and the lipoxygenase pathways and therefore inhibit the production of both leukotrienes and prostaglandins.

The Lipoxygenase Pathway In the lipoxygenase pathway, 5-lipoxygenase (produced by neutrophils) forms an active enzyme complex, 5-hydroxyeicosatetraenoic acid (5-HETE), a chemotactic agent, or a family of compounds called the **leukotrienes.** Leukotriene B$_4$ (LTB$_4$) is responsible for neutrophil chemotaxis. Other leukotrienes (LTC$_4$, LTD$_4$, and LTE$_4$) are involved in vasoconstriction, bronchospasm, and increased vascular permeability.

Clinical Correlation **Preeclampsia** is a multisystem disorder affecting 4% to 5% of all pregnancies. It is characterized by hypertension, proteinuria, and edema. Preeclampsia typically manifests after 20 weeks of gestation and affects nulliparas more commonly than multiparas. Preeclampsia

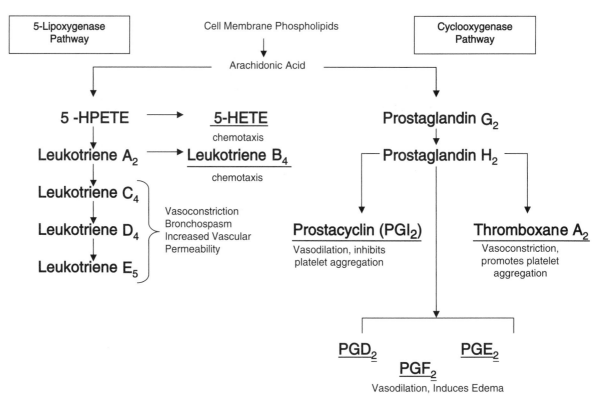

Figure 10-1 AA metabolites and their roles in inflammation.

can also affect maternal renal, cerebral, hepatic, and clotting functions likely as a result of abnormal blood vessel permeability and reactivity and platelet function.

The etiology of preeclampsia is not fully understood. Because the disease resembles and has many of the complications seen in systemic lupus erythematosus (SLE), it has been hypothesized that preeclampsia is caused by an immune response, possibly to paternal antigens on the trophoblastic tissue. Likely involved is an imbalance of thromboxane/prostacyclin as a result of deficient intravascular production of prostacyclin (vasodilation) and excessive production of thromboxane (favoring vasoconstriction and platelet aggregation). The clinical sequelae of this imbalance includes hypertension and renal damage (leading to proteinuria). These observations have led to the hypothesis that antiplatelet agents (low-dose aspirin) might prevent or delay the onset of preeclampsia.

Case Conclusion The patient is diagnosed with preeclampsia, admitted to labor and delivery, and placed on magnesium sulfate therapy for seizure prophylaxis (eclampsia). Because the only cure for preeclampsia is delivery, the decision is made to induce labor. Labor progresses smoothly, and the patient's BP and proteinuria remain stable. She delivers a 7-pound 5-ounce baby boy and is treated with magnesium sulfate for an additional 24 hours. Postpartum she and the baby do well and her BP returns to baseline.

Thumbnail: Eicosanoid Synthesis

Enzyme	Products	Action	Inhibitors
COX	Prostaglandins Thromboxane	Vasodilation, fever, pain Vasoconstriction, platelet aggregation	Aspirin, NSAIDs, COX inhibitors
Lipoxygenase	Leukotrienes	Increased vascular permeability	Corticosteroids

Key Points

▶ Eicosanoids (prostaglandins, thromboxanes, and leukotrienes) are 20-carbon amino acids produced from fatty acids released from membrane phospholipids.

▶ The precursor to eicosanoid synthesis is AA.

▶ AA metabolism proceeds by one of two major pathways named after the enzymes that initiate the reactions: the **COX pathway** and the **lipoxygenase pathway.**

▶ Glucocorticoids are powerful anti-inflammatory agents that act to inhibit the release of AA from membrane phospholipids.

▶ Aspirin and NSAIDs, such as indomethacin, ibuprofen, and COX inhibitors, inhibit COX and therefore inhibit prostaglandin synthesis.

Questions

1. Recent studies suggest that low-dose aspirin may prevent or delay the onset of preeclampsia. The probable mechanism is which of the following?

   A. Aspirin inhibits COX, which in turn inhibits the formation of prostacyclin, a potent vasoconstrictor and platelet aggregator.

   B. Aspirin inhibits COX, which in turn inhibits the formation of thromboxane, a potent vasodilator.

   C. Aspirin inhibits COX, which in turn inhibits the formation of leukotrienes, potent vasodilators.

   D. Aspirin inhibits COX, which in turn inhibits the formation of thromboxane, a potent vasoconstrictor and platelet aggregator.

   E. Aspirin inhibits COX, which in turn inhibits the formation of prostacyclin, a potent vasodilator.

2. _____, which is inhibited by _____, is required for the production of prostaglandins.

   A. COX, acetaminophen
   B. Lipoxygenase, aspirin
   C. COX, ibuprofen
   D. Lipoxygenase, indomethacin
   E. COX, terbutaline

HPI: EL is a 22-year-old woman who is concerned about her family history of blood clots. Her 19-year-old brother died last year of a stroke, and she had heard on TV that some blood-clotting diseases can run in families. EL has never had a stroke or blood clot. She is nearsighted but otherwise enjoys good health. She had a hard time in school, and throughout high school, she was in a special education program. She states that her behavior is sometimes erratic, and that last summer she was admitted overnight to a psychiatric unit because of "psychosis." Further review of family history does not reveal any other family member with a history of thromboembolic events. EL has an additional sister who is 25 years old and who finished college. Both of her parents are healthy in their late 50s and of average stature.

PE: Height 5'11" Weight 125 pounds. Appearance tall, slender, young woman with long skinny fingers. HEENT exam is notable for poor visual acuity and anterior displacement of the lens. She has mild kyphoscoliosis and pectus excavatum chest deformity. Cardiopulmonary exam is unremarkable.

Labs: CBC count shows platelets within normal limits; prothrombin time (PT), international normalized ratio (INR), partial thromboplastin time (PTT) within normal limits; factor V Leiden, methylenetetrahydrofolate reductase (MTHFR), and G20210A prothrombin molecular studies negative for any mutations; protein C, protein S deficiency negative; serum amino acids show elevated methionine and homocysteine, as well as low cysteine.

Thought Questions

- What is the diagnosis? How is the diagnosis made?

- What is the metabolic defect?

- What are the different strategies to correct the metabolic defect?

- Are there other disease states associated with elevated homocysteine levels?

Basic Science Review and Discussion

Homocystinuria is an AR inborn error of metabolism (IEM) characterized by the **accumulation of homocysteine, which may lead to ocular, musculoskeletal, central nervous system (CNS), and vascular manifestations.** Newborn screening for homocystinuria is possible, although not all state programs screen for this potentially treatable condition. Newborns appear normal, and early symptoms, if present, are vague. Visual problems may lead to diagnosis if the child is discovered on exam to have **dislocated lenses and myopia.** Displacement of the lens into the anterior chamber is highly suggestive of homocystinuria. **Musculoskeletal manifestations** include tall stature, thin body habitus, long skinny fingers, and pectus excavatum, as well as kyphoscoliosis. **Thromboembolic complications** occur in roughly 25% of patients by age 15 years if untreated. **Some degree of mental retardation** is usually seen, but some affected people have normal IQs. When mental retardation is present, it is generally progressive if left untreated. Psychiatric disease can also result; for example, psychoses.

Metabolic Defect Homocystinuria is due to cystathionine β-synthase (CBS) deficiency. **CBS** is an enzyme involved at the branching point between trans-sulfuration and remethylation in methionine degradation. Most of the homocysteine is converted to cystathionine and much less is remethylated back to methionine. However, in homocystinuria, the inactivity of CBS prevents homocysteine from trans-sulfuration to cystathionine and diverts it via remethylation to methionine. Consequently, there is elevated methionine and homocysteine, as well as low or absent cysteine. Diagnosis is confirmed by the detection of low levels of CBS on culture fibroblasts. Once the diagnosis is established, a therapeutic trial with vitamin B_6 (cofactor of CBS) should be done. Fifty percent of patients respond to vitamin B_6, some with full correction of the metabolic imbalance. Nutritional therapy with reduced amounts of methionine is necessary for all pyridoxine non-responders and partial responders. Betaine, a methyl group donor that lowers homocysteine levels by remethylating homocysteine to methionine, is also helpful in these vitamin B_6 non-responder patients.

Hyperhomocysteinemia and Vascular Disease Elevations of homocysteine can be a result of IEMs such as CBS deficiency but may also arise in common states like folate deficiency or B_{12} deficiency that impair remethylation. Folate and B_{12} are cofactors required in the one-carbon transfer reactions. There has been a well-established association between elevated homocysteine levels and vascular disease, in the coronary, carotid, and peripheral circulation. The mechanism by which this occurs is not fully understood, and whether interventions that decrease homocysteine levels can prevent the occurrence of these complications is not currently known.

Case Conclusion Homocystinuria is suspected, so a skin biopsy is performed for fibroblast culture, which shows no detectable CBS activity, confirming the diagnosis. EL then undergoes a trial of pyridoxine, showing marked metabolic improvement with normalization of homocysteine levels in plasma. Subjectively, EL says she feels better and has not had any more drastic mood changes. Because she has had a complete response to pyridoxine, there is no need for diet modifications.

Thumbnail: Homocystinuria

Trans-sulfuration Pathway Showing Key Enzymes, Cofactors, and Rate-limiting Steps

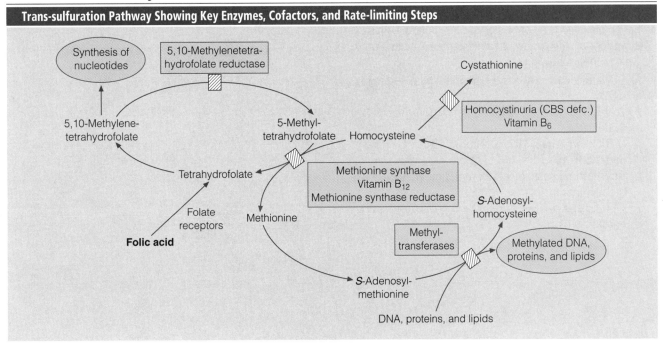

Key Points

▸ Features: ectopia lentis, tall and thin, mental retardation, thromboembolism

▸ Metabolic defect: elevated homocysteine, methionine, low cysteine level resulting from CBS deficiency

▸ Treatment: vitamin B_6; diet and betaine for partial or non-responders to vitamin B_6 treatment

Questions

1. A 26-year-old man presents to the ED with severe chest pain. He is tall and slender, and he has dislocation of the lens and a pectus carinatum deformity. What is the molecular basis for the underlying disorder?

   A. Fibrillin gene mutation
   B. CBS deficiency
   C. Drug abuse
   D. MTHFR mutations
   E. None of the above

2. During routine checkup, Mr. Smith, a 65-year-old patient, has an elevated level of homocysteine in plasma. Plasma elevations of homocysteine have been associated with which of the following?

   A. Dementia, coronary disease, neural tube defects (NTDs)
   B. Protein C deficiency, folic acid deficiency, vitamin B_6 deficiency
   C. MTHFR mutations, CBS mutations, factor V Leiden mutations
   D. Dolichostenomelia, mental retardation, normal methionine
   E. Cleft lip and palate, neural tube defects, holoprosencephaly

3. A 4-year-old child with displacement of the lens and mild developmental delays is brought to your office. You suspect homocystinuria. Of the following, which would you not expect to find?

   A. Arachnodactyly
   B. Low CBS activity in cultured fibroblast
   C. Elevated methionine and homocysteine in plasma
   D. Positive cyanide nitroprusside test
   E. Increased levels of phenylalanine in serum

HPI: PF, a 7-day-old infant, is brought to her pediatrician by her parents after receiving a call from the State Lab Newborn Screening Division. Her heel-stick dried blood spot is suspicious for phenylketonuria (PKU). Her mother tells you that PF was born via normal spontaneous vaginal delivery (NSVD) at term after an uncomplicated pregnancy. Her birth weight was 3.5 kg, height 51 cm, and head circumference 50 cm, all near the fiftieth percentile. She was discharged from the hospital on her second day of life, along with her mother. PF is being breast-fed exclusively. Both parents are quick to assert that she seems perfectly normal, and that she is no different from her two older siblings at the same age. They are terribly worried though because they read that PKU could cause mental retardation.

PE: Detailed exam reveals a perfectly normal 1-week-old infant.

Labs: Blood work was ordered by the State Lab. Serum amino acid tests show marked hyperphenylalaninemia (phenylalanine > 360 μmol/L), mild decrease in tyrosine.

Thought Questions

- What is the outcome of untreated and treated PKU?

- What is the metabolic defect in PKU?

- What is the molecular basis of this disorder?

Basic Science Review and Discussion

Initially recognized in mentally retarded adults who had high concentrations of phenylpyruvic acid in the urine, PKU is a classic example of an **inborn error of metabolism (IEM)** and has a successful history in terms of the prevention of mental retardation in affected individuals with PKU.

Natural History of Untreated PKU   Children with PKU, if untreated, are severely mentally retarded and have hypopigmentation and neurologic symptoms. Neurologic symptoms include hypertonicity, irritability, hyperactivity, and occasionally seizures. The mental retardation and other neurologic manifestations in PKU are thought to result from the accumulation of excessive amounts of phenylalanine and its derivatives. High levels of phenylalanine are toxic to the brain in experimental models and in humans. The hypopigmentation of skin and hair occurs because of the competitive inhibition of tyrosine hydroxylase by high levels of phenylalanine.

Results of Patients Treated for PKU   With accurate diagnosis and identification of PKU in the newborn period, and with initiation of a phenylalanine-restricted diet, children with PKU can develop normally. Phenylalanine is an essential amino acid, so it cannot be completely eliminated from the diet. Blood phenylalanine levels must be carefully monitored, particularly during the first 5 years of life, but continuation of the phenylalanine-restricted diet should be lifelong. Patients with PKU who go off the diet as teenagers or adults, though not mentally retarded, may develop neurologic symptoms such as irritability, agitated behavior, and difficulty in concentration. Women with PKU, if not under optimal metabolic control, are at risk of having mentally retarded offspring (maternal PKU syndrome).

Biochemistry and Molecular Basis   The enzyme responsible for the conversion of phenylalanine to tyrosine, phenylalanine hydroxylase (PAH), is deficient in PKU. This "enzymatic block" leads to the accumulation of phenylalanine and its metabolites (phenylpyruvic acid and phenylacetic acid, which are excreted in the urine), which are toxic to the brain. The levels in blood of tyrosine (the end product of PAH) are low, as anticipated. This decrease in tyrosine, in addition to the competitive inhibition of tyrosinase by the hyperphenylalaninemia, the enzyme that converts dopa to melanin (see Thumbnail: Phenylketonuria), is responsible for the hypopigmentation of untreated patients with PKU. There are many different mutations of the PAH gene, most of which are base substitutions found in exons 6 through 12. No single mutation seems to be predominant, and more than 70 have been identified. The frequency of PKU is about 1 in 10,000 newborns of western European descent and is lower in other populations.

Case Conclusion   PF was immediately placed on a phenyl-restricted diet. She was bottle-fed with a special formula until age 1 year and then gradually advanced to low-protein foods and continued to take her special phenyl-free formula. For years, she was followed at the metabolic clinic in her region. She tested in the high end of normal in all of her periodic neuropsychologic tests. As a teenager, PF had difficulty with compliance with her diet and went through some rough times at school. Fortunately, with lots of support from her parents and staff, she has been back on her diet fully. She is now 25 years old and thinking about having children.

Thumbnail: Phenylketonuria

Phenylalanine, Tyrosine, Dopa Pathway

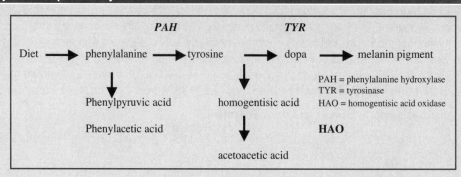

Key Points

▶ A block in a metabolic pathway leads to accumulation of intermediaries and/or deficiency of the end product.

▶ Several IEMs can be detected by newborn screening and successfully treated by dietary restriction, supplementation, or enzyme replacement.

▶ Most IEMs are AR. Most IEMs can be detected prenatally by either functional assays or DNA testing.

Questions

1. PF is now 10 weeks pregnant. Her fetus is at risk of mental retardation if which of the following is true?

   A. Her fetus is homozygous for the PAH mutation

   B. High levels of phenylalanine in maternal serum, independent of fetal PAH genotype

   C. Normal levels of tyrosine and normal levels of phenylalanine in maternal serum

   D. Low levels of phenylalanine in maternal serum, homozygous fetus for the PAH mutation

   E. The father is a carrier of the PAH mutation that is passed on to the fetus

2. A couple who has a 5-year-old son with PKU is interested in a prenatal diagnosis. Their son has classic PKU, but only one mutant allele was identified on DNA testing. Prenatal diagnosis is possible by means of which of the following?

   A. Liver biopsy of the fetus

   B. Is not possible because only one mutation was identified on the child with PKU

   C. Amniocentesis measuring PAH activity from amniocytes

   D. Linkage of the mutant allele using restriction fragment length polymorphisms (RFLPs) by means of chorionic villus sampling (CVS) or amniocentesis

   E. DNA testing of the fetus for mutations of PAH using CVS

3. A 10-day-old male infant in the neonatal ICU (NICU) has jaundice, hepatomegaly, and sepsis caused by a gram-negative rod. On review of the family history, you learn that his older sister had a similar course as a newborn and later developed cirrhosis of the liver and cataracts. The most likely diagnosis is which of the following?

   A. Homocystinuria

   B. Maple syrup urine disease

   C. Galactosemia

   D. Tyrosinemia

   E. Biotinidase deficiency

HPI: BG is a 5-month-old boy whose care is being transferred to you from a family physician in rural Minnesota. BG's mother presented late to prenatal care and received a formal sonogram at 29 weeks. The scan was remarkable for limb shortening and mild bowing of the long bones. BG was delivered by an uncomplicated spontaneous vaginally delivery at term. His infant course has been notable for mild growth retardation and a fracture of the left humerus at 4 months of age.

PE: His scleras are blue. His cardiovascular and pulmonary exams show no abnormalities. His abdominal exam reveals a small umbilical hernia. His extremities are short and bowed, and he has hyperextensible joints. His skin is thin and translucent, and there are multiple bruises on his body. Although there has been suspicion of child abuse, the referring physician assures you that is not the case. Upon questioning his mother, you discover that other family members have had similar problems as BG.

Thought Questions

■ What is osteogenesis imperfecta (OI)?

■ What connective tissue component is defective in this disease? What types of genetic errors lead to this disease?

■ Describe how collagen is made. Where in the synthesis pathway is collagen affected in this disorder?

Basic Science Review and Discussion

OI is a group of inherited diseases caused by abnormalities in type I collagen. These defects in collagen lead to increased susceptibility to bone fractures and skeletal deformities. There are four types of OI with increased fracturability as the common feature. Type II is not compatible with life. Type I is the most common form and is the focus of this review.

Collagen Synthesis   Let's first review collagen synthesis. Collagen consists of a family of fibrous proteins that are ubiquitous. It has a distinct feature of forming insoluble fibers of high tensile strength. In general, collagen is made of three polypeptide chains to form the basic unit called tropocollagen. The different combinations of polypeptide chains that make up the tropocollagen are what differentiates the types of collagen. For instance, type I collagen consists of two chains of $\alpha 1$(I) and one $\alpha 2$(I), whereas type II collagen contains three of the same polypeptides $\alpha 1$(II).

Collagen has many unique features. First, it has a unique composition of amino acids and sequence. There is a high proportion of glycine when compared with other proteins. Approximately one third of collagen is glycine; this is due to its regularity of the amino acid sequence, with glycine appearing as nearly every third amino acid. Proline is also present in high concentration. Hydroxylysine and hydroxy-proline, two forms of amino acids found in few other proteins, are abundant in collagen. Of note, the regularity

of the amino acid sequence is also unique to collagen. Globular proteins do not exhibit this feature. The triple strands of collagen form a helical rod that is 300 nm long and 1.5 nm in diameter and are hydrogen bonded. The hydrogen donor is from the amino group of the glycine residue, and the hydrogen-accepting group is the CO group from the other chains. It has been determined that glycine is critical as every third amino acid because of its small size, allowing it to fit in an interior position in the helix. Post-translational modifications, such as hydroxylation of proline and lysine, aid in increasing the stability of collagen.

The synthesis of collagen occurs first as procollagen, a precursor form that consists of the sequences for the tropocollagen and additional segments at the amino-terminal and carboxy-terminal (C-terminus). These end sequences, called propeptides, are different in composition from the tropocollagen, and they are linked to one another by disulfide bonds. They serve to prevent the premature formation of collagen fibers. Procollagen is synthesized in cells, where it undergoes post-translational modifications that include the hydroxylation of proline and lysine and the addition of carbohydrate units to the hydroxylysine residues. After these modifications they are secreted to the extracellular space. Once outside the cell, procollagen peptidases cleave the propeptide ends, allowing tropocollagens to come together to form a staggered array, which results in the formation of a collagen fiber. The formation of covalent cross-links between the tropocollagen molecules at lysine and hydroxylysine residues serve to further strengthen the collagen fiber.

Gene Mutations of OI   More than 50 mutations affect type I collagen synthesis leading to OI. Most patients with type I OI have a severely impaired production of type I collagen. Most of the time, it is due to an error in the pro$\alpha 1$(I) chain.

The mutations seen so far are those that interfere with intact messenger RNA (mRNA) synthesis such as promoter mutations or splicing mutations that ultimately lead to half the quantity of normal type I collagen. Other mutations lead to an abnormal procollagen quantity that affects the maturation of procollagen into a normal collagen fibril. In these cases, mutations that occur in the C-terminus can be disruptive by preventing the propagation of the triple helix formation. Post-translational modifications still occur in the remaining portion of the triple helix, distal to the mutation, but are overmodified, thereby impairing its secretion from the cell. These fibrils are abnormal and unstable, and their numbers are reduced by increased degradation. Clinically, this results in bone with abnormal collagen fibrils, and the reduction in the number of fibrils causes poor bone mineralization.

The mutations leading to OI are mostly **autosomal dominant,** but a few autosomal recessive forms do exist. A milder phenotype is seen when the consequence of the mutation is the reduction of normal type I collagen. The more severe forms occur when the mutation affects a type of procollagen and its ability to interact with other procollagens to form the collagen fibril. For example, if there were a mutation in one of the proα1(I) alleles, it would impair the contribution of normal proα1(I) and proα2(I) alleles because of the polymeric nature of collagen. This mutation in the proα1(I) allele is called a dominant negative allele and is one example of how the mutation in a multimeric protein can lead to a dominant phenotype.

Case Conclusion BG was diagnosed with OI type III. He presents to you many times during his early years with fractures. You recommend that he see a physical therapist to help with his motor development and ambulation. He starts early with dental care, given that individuals with OI have problems with dentition. You discuss with his parents that no cure is available, although there are bone-rodding procedures that help strengthen and prevent deformities of the long bones.

Thumbnail: Collagen Synthesis

Type	Phenotype	Biochemical defect	Gene defect
Type I	Mildest and most common Bone predisposed to fractures Normal to near-normal height Loose joints, low muscle tone Scleras blue, gray, or purple tint Bone deformities minimal Brittle teeth possible Hearing loss possible	Collagen normal but less	Null alleles that impair production, such as those that interfere with mRNA synthesis
Type II	Perinatal lethal Most severe form Numerous fractures Severe bone deformity Small stature Underdeveloped lungs	Collagen made is abnormal	Missense mutation in glycine codons of the genes for α1 and α2 chains
Type III	Bone predisposed to fracture Short stature Loose joints, poor muscle tone Barrel-shaped rib cage Curved spine Respiratory difficulties Severe bone deformities Brittle teeth possible Hearing loss possible	Collagen made is abnormal	Missense mutation in glycine codons of the genes for α1 and α2 chains
Type IV	Severity between types I and III Bones fracture easily Shorter than average stature Scleras white/near white Mild to moderate deformities Spinal curvature Barrel-shaped rib cage Brittle teeth possible Hearing loss possible	Collagen made is abnormal	Missense mutation in glycine codons of the genes for α1 and α2 chains Exon-skipping mutation in 5′ end of the α2 gene

Key Points

▶ Collagen consists of three polypeptide chains (pro-collagen) to form the basic structural unit called tropocollagen.

▶ Collagen has an unusual amino acid composition, with a high amount of glycine, occurring in every third position, a high amount of proline, and the presence of hydroxylysine and hydroxyproline, which are rare in other proteins.

▶ The procollagen undergoes post-translational modifications, including hydroxylation of specific proline and lysine and then glycosylation of hydroxylysine, and then procollagen is cleaved once outside of the cell.

▶ The tensile strength of collagen is dependent on the helical nature of collagen, the hydroxylation of proline, the amount of glycosylation, and the cross-linking between collagen fibers at lysine and hydroxylysine.

▶ OI is a group of inherited, primarily AD diseases that is characterized by a defect in type I collagen synthesis. There are four types, but type I is the most common. Type II is the lethal form.

▶ Dominant negative allele is when there is a mutation in one polypeptide of a multimeric protein that disrupts the function of the whole protein despite normal expression of the other proteins in multimeric protein. Therefore, the one mutation results in a dominant phenotype.

Questions

1. Scurvy is a connective tissue disease caused by a deficiency of ascorbic acid (vitamin C). In the 1500s, sailors lacking ascorbic acid in their diet would suffer from poor healing, bleeding gums, and easy bruising. It was not until 1753 when a Scottish physician observed that scurvy could be prevented when sailors had access to a diet with fresh fruits and vegetables. What is the role of ascorbic acid in collagen synthesis?

   A. To serve as a cofactor to lysyl oxidase, which is necessary for cross-linking adjacent tropocollagen molecules

   B. To serve as a cofactor to procollagen peptidase in the excision of the propeptides before secretion

   C. To maintain prolyl hydroxylase in the active form by keeping its iron atom in the reduced ferrous state

   D. To maintain lysyl hydroxylase in the active form by keeping its iron atom in the reduced ferrous state

   E. To inhibit the action of collagenase and prevent early degradation of the collagen molecule

2. More than 50 mutations can affect type I collagen synthesis, leading to OI. Which of the following mutations causes the most severe form of type I OI?

   A. A mutation in the proα1(I) allele that leads to an absence of its synthesis from that allele

   B. A mutation in the proα2(I) allele that leads to a reduction of type I collagen molecules

   C. A missense mutation in the proα1(I) allele that affects the triple helix formation of collagen, resulting in abnormal collagen molecules

   D. Missense mutations in the glycine codons of the α1 and α2 chains of type I collagen

   E. Exon skipping in the 5′ end of the α2 chain gene.

3. Collagen is unique because of which of the following?

   A. It has a high proline concentration, with one in every third position.

   B. It contains exogenous hydroxyproline that is incorporated into the amino acid sequence.

   C. The proline molecule is critical because it is small and is able to fit in the interior position of the helical strand.

   D. It has a very regular sequence with the frequent recurrence of glycine-proline-hydroxyproline.

   E. Most lysine residues are converted to hydroxylysine by lysyl hydroxylase.

HPI: JT is a 7-month-old female brought in by her mother with her eighth bad cold. The infant has had symptoms of an upper respiratory tract infection for 2 days. Her mother reports that JT has had many colds, but this time she is particularly concerned because it is associated with a high fever and that JT seems much sicker. The infant's medical history is significant for recurrent upper respiratory tract infections and thrush, as well as a recent "bout of the stomach flu." Of note, the infant's pediatrician is concerned about her growth because she has fallen off her growth curve, from the sixty-eighth percentile at birth down to the twenty-second percentile at her 6-month well-baby visit. Her vital signs are taken, and she is noted to be febrile with a temperature of 39°C, tachycardic, with an oxygen saturation (O_2 Sat) of 92% on room air.

PE: She is irritable and her lung exam is remarkable for coarse breath sounds and consolidation at the right base.

Labs: A CBC count is significant for a normal white blood cell (WBC) count but a low lymphocyte count of 0.5 cell/μL. A chest x-ray reveals consolidation in the right lower lobe, consistent with pneumonia.

Thought Questions

- What cell type is affected in severe combined immunodeficiency (SCID) syndrome?

- Which biochemical and cellular pathways are defective in SCID?

- How are purines and pyrimidines made? What regulatory mechanisms are involved in their biosynthesis? How is cell proliferation affected by an alteration in these synthetic pathways?

Basic Science Review and Discussion

SCID syndrome is a heterogeneous disorder caused by defects in T-cell function and abnormal antibody-mediated immunity.

Approximately 50% of cases of SCID are due to a deficiency of adenosine deaminase (ADA), which is transmitted through an AR mode of inheritance. ADA catalyzes the deamination of adenosine and deoxyadenosine to inosine and 2'-deoxyinosine. In the absence of ADA, there is an accumulation of deoxyadenosine and deoxy-ATP, which becomes toxic to lymphocytes. The inhibition of ribonucleotide reductase and transmethylation reactions by the metabolites ultimately leads to a block in DNA synthesis. A deficiency in purine nucleoside phosphorylase, an enzyme involved in purine catabolism, also results in the accumulation of toxic metabolites and causes SCID in a similar manner as ADA deficiency (see Thumbnail: Purine Metabolism). Defects in interleukin-2 (IL-2) or its receptor and in T-cell receptor (TCR) signaling are other causes of SCID.

Purine Synthesis Purines are made from both a de novo pathway and a salvage reaction. In the de novo pathway, the purine ring is built using various precursor molecules. These include amino acids, tetrahydrofolate (THF) derivatives, and CO_2. The backbone of the ring is formed on a ribose phosphate that is donated by 5-phosphoribosyl-1-pyrophosphate (PRPP), and the formation of 5-phosphoribosylamine from PRPP and glutamine serves as the committed step into this pathway. The following steps involve the addition of a glycine, formylation, amination, and then ring closure, resulting in the 5-aminoimidazole ribonucleotide. Next, there is the addition of the CO_2, a formyl group, and the nitrogen from aspartate. This ring is then closed to yield inosine monophosphate (IMP), which contains a completed purine ring. IMP then goes on to form adenylate (i.e., AMP) and guanylate (i.e., GMP). The salvage reaction recycles the purine bases that are hydrolyzed in the degradation of nucleic acids and nucleotides. Here, the preformed purine base combines with the ribose from PRPP to create a purine nucleotide. The biosynthesis of purines is regulated by feedback inhibition of enzymes PRPP synthetase and glutamine PRPP aminotransferase by IMP, AMP, and GMP.

Purine Degradation The common end product of all purine degradation is uric acid. GTP is converted to guanosine by the enzyme nucleotidase. The bond to ribose phosphate is broken next, leaving guanine, which is converted to xanthine by guanase. Xanthine oxidase converts xanthine to uric acid. ATP is either broken down to adenosine and then to inosine by ADA or converted initially to IMP by AMP deaminase, which is then converted to inosine. Inosine is converted to hypoxanthine by purine nucleotide phosphorylase. Xanthine oxidase then creates xanthine from hypoxanthine and then uric acid from xanthine. IMP degradation begins by conversion to inosine by nucleotidase and continues down the same pathway as ATP.

Pyrimidine Synthesis Pyrimidine synthesis differs from purine synthesis primarily in that the ribose molecule is attached at the end, rather than being the first building block. Synthesis begins with glutamine and a bicarbonate becoming carbamoylphosphate catalyzed by carbamoyl-phosphate synthetase II (CPS-II). A glutamate is added to carbamoylphosphate to create *N*-carbamoylaspartate. This molecule releases a water molecule catalyzed by dihydro-orotase to create dihydro-orotate. Orotate is created by the dehydrogenase enzyme, which creates a double bond. At this point, the ribose phosphate is added by transferase, forming orotidylate. Feedback inhibition by pyrimidines also regulates their biosynthesis. The monophosphate, diphosphate, and triphosphate forms of the nucleosides are interconverted by kinases.

Pyrimidine Degradation   Pyrimidines are broken down to amino acids. The triphosphate molecules are converted to monophosphates. CMP is then converted to cytidine, and then uridine. Uridine monophosphate (UMP) is initially converted to uridine. Uridine then undergoes conversion to uracil, dihydrouracil, and eventually becomes β-alanine. Thymidine monophosphate (TMP) becomes thymine, dihydrothymine, and eventually β-aminoisobutyrate.

Deoxyribonucleotide Production   Deoxyribonucleotides are the precursors of DNA. They are formed by the reduction of ribonucleoside diphosphate by ribonucleotide reductase. Deoxythymidine monophosphate (dTMP) is formed by the methylation of deoxyuridine monophosphate (dUMP) by thymidylate synthase. The methyl group is donated by N^5,N^{10}-methylenetetrahydrofolate, which is then converted to dihydrofolate (DHF). Dihydrofolate reductase (DHFR) regenerates DHF to THF, its reduction with NADPH. Several chemotherapeutic agents, including methotrexate, inhibit the function of DHFR, which ultimately results in the inhibition of DNA synthesis and cell proliferation.

SCID   Patients with SCID most commonly present with serious and recurrent infections by the time they are 3 to 6 months of age. Common findings include failure to thrive and chronic respiratory tract, GI tract, or cutaneous infections. Infants can also have oral ulcers, oral esophageal candidiasis, severe varicella, and secretory diarrhea. Infections with opportunistic pathogens, such as *Pneumocystis carinii* or CMV, are indicative of an immunodeficiency. SCID is due to an abnormal development of T-cells and B-cells from the bone marrow stem cells. The thymus and peripheral lymphoid tissues have few or no lymphocytes. A low lymphocyte count of less than 1200 cells/μL is typical of SCID, although a normal count would not exclude it as a diagnosis

Thumbnail: Purine Metabolism

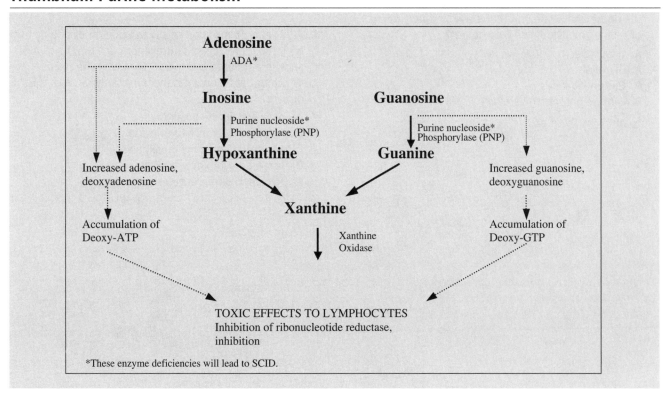

Key Points

▶ Purines are synthesized from amino acids, THF derivatives, and CO_2. In the de novo pathway, the purine ring is formed on a ribose phosphate (from the pentose phosphate pathway), and the salvage reaction uses free purine bases formed by the degradation of nucleic acids and nucleotides.

▶ Pyrimidines are synthesized from carbamoylphosphate and aspartate. The pyrimidine nucleotide is formed first by assembling the pyrimidine ring and then by linking it to a ribose phosphate.

▶ Deoxyribonucleotides are the precursors to DNA and are formed by the reduction of ribonucleosides by the enzyme ribonucleotide reductase.

▶ Uracil, which is found in RNA, is methylated by thymidylate synthase to form thymine, a component of DNA. The conversion of DHF to THF by DHFR is an essential step in DNA biosynthesis.

Questions

1. When considering patients with disruptions in purine synthesis, it is important to know what molecules are used. Which of the following is not a precursor in the synthesis of the purine ring?
   A. Aspartate
   B. CO_2
   C. THF derivatives
   D. Carbamoylphosphate
   E. Glycine

2. Which of the following is responsible for generation of the ribose phosphate unit that is used in the synthesis of purine and pyrimidine biosynthesis?
   A. Urea cycle
   B. Glycolysis
   C. Gluconeogenesis
   D. Pentose phosphate pathway
   E. Citric acid cycle

3. In patients with purine or pyrimidine synthesis problems, these disruptions can arise because of enzyme mutations that lead to dysfunctional enzymes, but also if enzymes do not respond to normal regulation. The critical enzymes in the biosynthesis of both purine and pyrimidine nucleotides are regulated by which of the following?
   A. Feedback inhibition
   B. Allosteric interaction
   C. Regulatory proteins
   D. Covalent modification
   E. Proteolytic activation

4. A 72-year-old man presents with acute onset of pain in his left big toe. It is so sensitive to touch that he cannot allow the sheet to touch it at night while he sleeps. Which of the following is the most likely cause of this disease?
   A. Increased purine breakdown
   B. Increased clearance of uric acid
   C. Increased pyrimidine breakdown
   D. Increased pyrimidine synthesis
   E. Decreased purine synthesis

HPI: This is the second visit of PW to the ED in the last month. She is a 19-year-old female who complains of intermittent abdominal pain and nausea for the last 2 days. She had a single episode of emesis, with no diarrhea. She also reports mild dysuria and frequency. She is on day 2 of her menses and has not been sexually active in the last 4 months. She is a junior in college, in the middle of final exams. She is quite anxious and has trouble concentrating. You review the records from the last visit and notice similar complaints, and overall a benign exam and unremarkable laboratory exams.

PE: Pulse 110; BP 120/68; RR 18; Afebrile
Young well-developed woman in no acute distress. Abdomen: mild diffuse tenderness to palpation, mildly distended, no guarding, no peritoneal signs. Unremarkable pelvic exam.

Labs: WBC count 9000/μL, hemoglobin concentration (Hgb) 10.2 g/dL, platelets 232/μL, normal smear

Na 141, K 4.5, CO_2 26, Cl 101, blood urea nitrogen (BUN) 12, creatinine (Cr) 0.6 mg/dL

Human chorionic gonadotropin (hCG) in urine: negative

Urinalysis (UA): Dark, port-wine color urine with specific gravity of 1.005

Thought Questions

- You suspect which diagnosis?
- How can you confirm the suspected diagnosis?
- What is the metabolic defect?

Basic Science Review and Discussion

Acute intermittent porphyria (AIP) is the most important of the hepatic porphyrias. AIP and other genetic porphyrias are unusual among enzyme deficiencies because they are manifested in the heterozygous state. AIP is an AD disorder characterized by a variety of other neuropathic symptoms. Between episodes, the patient is healthy. The most common symptom is abdominal pain, sometimes with constipation and/or diarrhea. Urinary symptoms are also common with dysuria, frequency, and urinary retention. Many other phenomena, including seizures, psychotic episodes, tachycardia, and hypertension, occur in acute attacks. Paresthesias and paralysis also occur, and death may result from respiratory tract paralysis. These attacks rarely occur before puberty. Attacks are more common in women, especially at the time of menses. Some women may benefit from drugs that inhibit ovulation. The acute attacks may be precipitated by drugs such as barbiturates and sulfonamides, alcohol, infection, inadequate nutrition, and hormonal changes.

Metabolic Defect Porphyrins are synthesized by a multistep reaction starting with succinyl-CoA and glycine. The first step of the reaction sequence is catalyzed by the enzyme δ-*aminolevulinate synthetase,* which is regulated through feedback inhibition by the ultimate end point of the sequence, heme. The chelation of iron in the final step produces heme, which is used as a prosthetic group in Hgb, myoglobin, catalase, peroxidase, and cytochrome *c.*

Several inherited disorders are associated with the porphyrin synthetic pathway. Most of these disorders, such as AIP, are inherited as ADs and affected individuals have 50% of the normal activity level of the affected enzyme. Most enzyme deficiency disorders are inherited as recessives, and heterozygotes with 50% activity do not manifest the phenotype. But the porphyrin pathway seems to have several rate-limiting steps so that a reduction of enzyme activity to 50% elicits an observable phenotype. Homozygotes are severely affected, but homozygosity is rare.

The basic biochemical defect in AIP is a reduction in the level of activity of porphobilinogen (PBG) deaminase. Enzyme activity in carriers of the mutant gene is reduced to approximately half the normal level in liver, fibroblasts, and RBCs. During or between acute attacks some patients with latent AIP intermittently excrete excess porphyrin precursors in the urine. The diagnosis is suspected by the presence of excessive amounts of aminolevulinic acid (ALA) and PBG in the urine. Ninety percent of patients with PBG deaminase deficiency are clinically unaffected. The acute attacks may be precipitated by a large number of drugs, some of which are known to induce the earlier rate-controlling step in heme synthesis, δ-ALA synthesis. Porphyrins may be formed in the urine from the precursors, turning the urine red or port wine, which may be a clue in the diagnosis.

Case Conclusion   Because of your high clinical suspicion, you initiate supportive treatment for an acute attack of por-phyria, providing high caloric intake and analgesic management with narcotics. The diagnosis is made by increased urinary δ-ALA and PBG in 24-hour urine and later confirmed by functional assay of erythrocyte PBG deaminase defi-ciency. You recommend to PW to wear a bracelet indicating her medical condition at all times.

Thumbnail: Acute Intermittent Porphyria

Heme Formation

Heme formation and rate-limiting steps.

	Enzyme	Porphyria	Frequency
1	ALA synthase	—	—
2	PBG synthase (ALA dehydratase)	PBG synthase deficiency	Unknown
3	PBG deaminase	AIP	1 to 2/100,000
4	Uroporphyrinogen III synthase	Congenital erythropoietic porphyria	<1/1,000,000
5	Uroporphyrinogen decarboxylase	Porphyria cutanea tarda	1/25,000
6	Coproporphyrinogen oxidase	Hereditary coproporphyria	1/250,000
7	Protoporphyrinogen oxidase	Variegate porphyria	1/250,000
8	Ferrochelatase	Erythropoietic protoporphyria	1/200,000

Key Points

- One of few AD IEMs
- Caused by erythrocyte PBG deaminase deficiency (exception: type II AIP)
- During acute attacks, increased δ-ALA and PBG in urine
- Attacks precipitated by drugs (e.g., barbiturates and sulfonamides), alcohol, infection, starvation, and hormonal changes

Questions

1. By chance, PW later marries AP, who is also affected by AIP. Of the following choices, which is the best answer?
   A. 50% chance of having a homozygous child with AIP, who would be severely affected
   B. 50% chance of having a child heterozygous for PBG deficiency, who may or may not be affected with AIP
   C. 25% chance of having a child heterozygous for AIP, who would be affected similar to the parents
   D. 50% chance of homozygous for PBG deficiency that would be severely affected
   E. 75% chance of having a heterozygous child, affected similarly to the parents

2. PW has another acute attack, but this time, it is further complicated by a seizure. Which medication(s) could most worsen her condition?
   A. Morphine
   B. Phenytoin
   C. Ibuprofen
   D. Carbamazepine
   E. Propanolol

> **HPI:** HA is an 18-month-old male infant who is brought to the ED by his parents. They note that he has had symptoms of a viral illness for the past 3 days, but today he began with increased vomiting and became uncooperative and combative. His mom says that he has gotten like this before when he gets sick, but this is the most violent he has become. Upon further history, they note that he has had episodes like this five or six times, and that during the last one, he was diagnosed with Reye's syndrome at age 15 months.
>
> **PE:** HA is febrile to 101.3°F, mildly tachycardic, and showing other signs of dehydration. On neurologic exam, you note that he is hyperreflexic and has mild asterixis and a positive Babinski's sign.
>
> **Labs:** CBC count and liver function tests (LFTs) return normal, except for an elevated ammonia level.

Thought Questions

- What genetic diagnoses should the ED doctor consider?
- What key findings help make this diagnosis?
- What are the key elements of the urea cycle?
- What are the common derangements of the urea cycle?

Basic Science Review and Discussion

The key finding in this patient's laboratory results is an elevated **ammonia** level. Interestingly, ammonia levels are not commonly ordered in routine work-ups of children, but they are ordered in this case because of the physical finding of **asterixis**, which is a flapping reflex of the hands when they are held out in front in a hyperextended position. Elevated ammonia levels are seen most commonly in the setting of liver failure, but this patient does not have liver function test abnormalities. Another way to see elevated ammonia levels is the hyperammonemia syndromes, such as CPS deficiency (type I hyperammonemia) or ornithine transcarbamoylase (OTC) deficiency (type II hyperammonemia), or other derangements of enzymes in the **urea cycle.** To better understand these deficiencies, we first need to understand the processes of the urea cycle.

The Urea Cycle   Twenty percent of nitrogenous waste can be excreted in the kidney, where **glutaminase** is responsible for converting excess glutamine from the liver to urine ammonium. However, about 80% of the excreted nitrogen is in the form of urea, which is also largely made in the liver, in a series of reactions that are distributed between the mitochondrial matrix and the cytosol. The series of reactions that form urea is known as the **urea cycle,** or the **Krebs-Henseleit cycle.**

Removal of Nitrogen from Amino Acids   The dominant reactions involved in removing amino acid nitrogen from the body are known as **transaminations.** This class of reactions funnels nitrogen from all free amino acids into a small number of compounds; then, either they are oxidatively deaminated, producing ammonia, or their amine groups are converted to urea by the urea cycle. The remaining carbon skeleton of these amino acids can then enter into carbohydrate metabolism either in gluconeogenesis or in the TCA cycle. Transaminations involve moving an α-amino group from a donor α-amino acid to the keto carbon of an acceptor α-keto acid. **Aminotransferases** catalyze these reactions and use pyridoxal phosphate as a cofactor.

Generation of Urea   The essential features of the urea cycle reactions and their metabolic regulation are as follows: Arginine from the diet or from protein breakdown is cleaved by the cytosolic enzyme **arginase,** generating urea and ornithine. In subsequent reactions of the urea cycle, a new urea residue is built on the ornithine, regenerating arginine and perpetuating the cycle (Figure 16-1). Because the urea cycle is cyclic, the first step is often arbitrarily chosen to begin with ornithine arising in the cytosol. Ornithine is transported to the mitochondrial matrix, where **OTC** catalyzes its condensation with carbamoylphosphate, producing citrulline. The energy for the reaction is provided by the high-energy anhydride of carbamoylphosphate. The product, citrulline, is then transported to the cytosol, where the remaining reactions of the cycle take place.

The synthesis of citrulline requires a prior activation of carbon and nitrogen as carbamoylphosphate. The activation step requires two equivalents of ATP and the mitochondrial matrix enzyme *CPS-I.* There are two CPSs: a mitochondrial enzyme (CPS-I), which forms carbamoylphosphate destined for inclusion in the urea cycle, and a cytosolic CPS (CPS-II), which is involved in pyrimidine nucleotide biosynthesis. CPS-I is positively regulated by the allosteric effector *N*-acetylglutamate, while the cytosolic enzyme is acetylglutamate independent. In a two-step reaction, catalyzed by cytosolic **argininosuccinate synthetase,** citrulline and aspartate are condensed to form argininosuccinate. The reaction involves the addition of AMP (from ATP) to the amido carbonyl of citrulline, forming an activated intermediate on the enzyme surface (AMP citrulline), and the subsequent addition of aspartate to form argininosuccinate.

Arginine and fumarate are produced from argininosuccinate by the cytosolic enzyme **argininosuccinate lyase** (also called **argininosuccinase**). In the final step of the cycle, **arginase** cleaves urea from aspartate, regenerating cytosolic ornithine, which can be transported to the mitochondrial matrix for another round of urea synthesis. The fumarate, generated via the action of **argininosuccinate lyase,** is reconverted to aspartate for use in the **argininosuccinate synthetase** reaction. This occurs through the actions of cytosolic versions of the TCA cycle enzymes, **fumarase** (which yields malate) and **malate dehydrogenase** (which yields oxaloacetate).

Bioenergetics Beginning and ending with **ornithine,** the reactions of the cycle consume three equivalents of ATP

and four high-energy nucleotide phosphates. Urea is the only new compound generated by the cycle; all other intermediates and reactants are recycled. The energy consumed in the production of urea is more than recovered by the release of energy formed during the synthesis of the urea cycle intermediates. Ammonia released during the glutamate dehydrogenase reaction is coupled to the formation of NADH. In addition, when fumarate is converted back to aspartate, the malate dehydrogenase reaction used to convert malate to oxaloacetate generates a mole of NADH. These two moles of NADH, thus, are oxidized in the mitochondria, yielding six moles of ATP.

Regulation of the Urea Cycle The urea cycle operates only to eliminate excess nitrogen. On high-protein diets, the

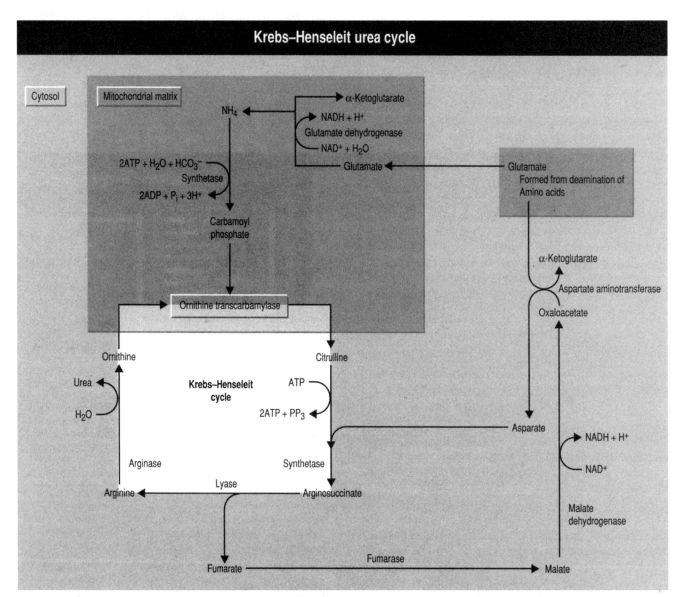

Figure 16-1 The principal steps of the urea cycle. The rectangle encloses the reactions that occur in the mitochondrion. (Reproduced with permission from Greenstein B. Medical Biochemistry at a Glance. Oxford: Blackwell Science, 1996.)

carbon skeletons of the amino acids are oxidized for energy or stored as fat and glycogen, but the amino nitrogen must be excreted. To facilitate this process, enzymes of the urea cycle are controlled at the gene level. With long-term changes in the quantity of dietary protein, there can be up to a 20-fold increase in the production of urea cycle enzymes. When dietary protein increases significantly, so do concomitant urea cycle enzymes. Under conditions of starvation, enzyme levels rise as proteins are degraded and amino acid carbon skeletons are used to provide energy, thus increasing the quantity of nitrogen that must be excreted. Short-term regulation of the cycle occurs principally at CPS-I, which is relatively inactive in the absence of its allosteric activator N-acetylglutamate. The steady-state concentration of N-acetylglutamate is set by the concentration of its components acetyl-CoA and glutamate and by arginine, which increases the activity of N-acetylglutamate synthetase.

Urea Cycle Defects A complete lack of any one of the enzymes of the urea cycle will result in death shortly after birth. However, deficiencies in each of the enzymes of the urea cycle, including N-acetylglutamate synthase, have been identified. These disorders are referred to as urea cycle disorders (UCDs). A common thread to most UCDs is hyperammonemia leading to ammonia intoxication. Deficiencies in arginase do not lead to symptomatic hyperammonemia as severe or as commonly as in the other UCDs. Clinical symptoms are most severe when the UCD is at the level of CPS-I.

Symptoms of UCDs usually present shortly after birth and include ataxia, convulsions, lethargy, poor feeding, and eventually coma and death if not recognized and treated properly. In fact, the mortality rate is 100% for UCDs that are left undiagnosed. In general, the treatment of UCDs have as common elements the reduction of protein in the diet, removal of excess ammonia, and replacement of intermediates missing from the urea cycle. Administration of levulose reduces ammonia through its action of acidifying the colon. Bacteria metabolize levulose to acidic by-products, which then promotes excretion of ammonia in the feces as ammonium ions, NH_4^+. Antibiotics can be administered to kill intestinal ammonia-producing bacteria. Dietary supplementation with arginine or citrulline can increase the rate of urea production in certain UCDs.

OTC deficiency is the most common of the UCDs. It is transmitted as an X-linked dominant disorder with males affected more strongly than females. It can present in infancy to early childhood. Episodes are usually instigated by periods of stress or a high-protein diet. Symptoms include vomiting, neurologic changes, ataxia, combativeness, and agitation. A hyperammonemic coma can evolve and if untreated and undiagnosed can lead to death. As far as development is concerned, these children will often be delayed and may have mild to moderate mental retardation. Specific diagnosis of OTC deficiency is made via laboratory findings during an acute exacerbation of symptoms finding hyperammonemia and elevated orotic acid secretion in the urine. This finding differentiates this disease from CPS deficiency, which may present identically. Prenatal diagnosis of OTC can be made via fetal liver biopsy, although there should be a prenatal genetic diagnosis, which can be done via amniocentesis, available soon.

Case Conclusion HA has elevated urine orotic acid levels, making the diagnosis. He is acutely treated with levulose, sodium benzoate, IV hydration, and a nonprotein diet supplemented with simple amino acids. He recovers in the hospital after several days and is discharged home into the care of his parents with this new diagnosis and advice about management of this disease. The family is scheduled for follow-up in 1 week with the geneticist who has seen them in the hospital.

Thumbnail: The Urea Cycle

Urea cycle disorder	Enzyme deficiency	Symptoms/comments
Type I hyperammonemia	CPS-I	1 to 3 days after birth, infant becomes lethargic, with vomiting, hypothermia, and hyperventilation; without measurement of serum ammonia levels and appropriate intervention, infant will die: treatment with arginine, which activates N-acetylglutamate synthetase
N-acetylglutamate synthetase	N-acetylglutamate synthetase	Severe hyperammonemia associated with deep coma, acidosis, recurrent diarrhea, ataxia, hypoglycemia, hyperornithinemia; treatment includes administration of carbamoylglutamate to activate CPS-I
Type II hyperammonemia	OTC	Most commonly occurring UCD; only X-linked UCD; ammonia and amino acids elevated in serum; increased serum orotic acid due to mitochondrial carbamoylphosphate entering cytosol and being incorporated into pyrimidine nucleotides, which leads to excess production and consequently excess catabolic products; treat with high-carbohydrate, low-protein diet, ammonia detoxification with sodium phenylacetate or sodium benzoate
Classic citrullinemia	Argininosuccinate synthetase	Episodic hyperammonemia, vomiting, lethargy, ataxia, seizures, eventual coma; treat with arginine administration to enhance citrulline excretion, also with sodium benzoate for ammonia detoxification
Argininosuccinic aciduria	Argininosuccinate lyase (argininosuccinase)	Episodic symptoms similar to classic citrullinemia; elevated plasma and cerebral spinal fluid (CSF) argininosuccinate; treat with arginine and sodium benzoate
Hyperargininemia	Arginase	Rare UCD; progressive spastic quadriplegia and mental retardation; ammonia and arginine high in CSF and serum; arginine, lysine, and ornithine high in urine; treatment includes diet of essential amino acids excluding arginine, low-protein diet

Key Points

▶ Nitrogenous waste is primarily excreted by the kidney, although only about 20% of it is converted to ammonium in the kidney.

▶ Eighty percent of nitrogenous waste is converted to urea primarily by the liver in the urea cycle.

▶ Short-term regulation of the urea cycle occurs at CPS-I, which is activated by N-acetylglutamate.

▶ N-acetylglutamate is increased by acetyl-CoA, glutamate, and arginine.

▶ Long-term regulation of the urea cycle is primarily at the gene level that up-regulates with increases in dietary protein and starvation.

▶ Without the normal functioning of the urea cycle, there is buildup of nitrogenous waste, which can cause the disease mentioned in the thumbnail.

Questions

1. The key regulatory step in the urea cycle is catalyzed by which of the following?
   - A. CPS-I
   - B. N-acetylglutamate synthetase
   - C. OTC
   - D. Argininosuccinate synthetase
   - E. Arginase

2. The symptoms seen in patients with UCDs are primarily secondary to what?
   - A. Excess serum urea
   - B. Excess plasma orotic acid
   - C. Hyperammonemia
   - D. Hypoammonemia
   - E. Decreased renal function

> **HPI:**   GH is a 16-year-old previously healthy female brought to the ED by her mother after being ill for 3 days. She reports initially having some dysuria but did not seek treatment. Her urinary symptoms worsened over the next two days. On the day of presentation, she reports having a fever, with a temperature of 38.9°C, chills, lack of appetite, nausea, vomiting, lethargy, and abdominal pain. The only significant additional information in the review of symptoms is that she has had a 15-pound weight loss over the last 2 months. She has also been more thirsty, drinking more water, and urinating much more frequently both during the day and at night over the last few months. Her medical history is unremarkable, but her family history is notable for diabetes, thyroid disease, and rheumatoid arthritis.
>
> **PE:**   She is febrile to 38.5°C, tachycardic to the 110s, and hypotensive at 88/49 mm Hg but shows no remarkable signs of dehydration and tenderness in the epigastric, suprapubic region, and over the left costovertebral angle.
>
> **Labs:**   WBC count 28,000/μL, metabolic acidosis with an anion gap, random serum glucose 452 mg/dL, UA significant for a urinary tract infection (UTI)

Thought Questions

- What do you suspect is going on with this patient?

- What is diabetes mellitus? What is the cause of type I diabetes mellitus?

- How does insulin signaling occur? What are some intracellular mediators regulating the downstream effects of insulin?

Basic Review and Discussion

Type I diabetes mellitus is a chronic disease characterized by the relative paucity of insulin and hyperglycemia due to the inability of the pancreas to secrete insulin. Most commonly, this is due to the destruction of the beta cells of the pancreas, the insulin-secreting cells, by an autoimmune process. It has been shown that individuals have a genetic susceptibility for getting type I diabetes. These individuals are exposed to a virus, environmental agent, or toxin that precipitates an immunologic destruction of the beta cells. After 80% to 90% of the beta cells are destroyed, an individual will become diabetic. In this review, we primarily focus on the insulin signaling and the regulators of this pathway.

Insulin is a **polypeptide hormone** that is integral in the **regulation of metabolic processes.** It functions to promote **anabolic processes** and inhibits catabolic processes in the muscle, liver, and fatty tissues. The action of insulin is to **increase the synthetic rates of glycogen, fatty acids, and proteins.** It promotes the entry of glucose and other sugars, as well as amino acids, into muscle and fat cells. It acts to prevent catabolism such as the breakdown of fat and glycogen, and it decreases gluconeogenesis.

Insulin is first produced as **preproinsulin** and is directed to the endoplasmic reticulum by the signal sequence, the 19-residue sequence at the amino-terminal. While in the lumen of the endoplasmic reticulum, it is **converted** into **proinsulin** by cleavage of the signal sequence. The proinsulin is transported to the Golgi complex and then to secretory granules. It is within the secretory granules that the connecting peptide, also known as the **C-peptide,** is cleaved. This mature form of insulin is stored in the secretory granules and is secreted when the granules fuse with the plasma membrane of the beta cell.

Insulin Signaling   Insulin acts by binding to insulin receptors on the surface of target cells. The **insulin receptor is an integral membrane glycoprotein** and consists of two α chains and two β chains, connected by three disulfide bonds. The α chains are found extracellularly, and the β chains traverse the plasma membrane. Two forms of the insulin receptor exist and are products of alternate MRNA splicing of exon 11 of the proreceptor transcript. The two transcripts differ in 12 amino acids. The final receptors have also been shown to differ in their ability to mediate insulin action.

Once insulin binds to this cognate receptor on the α chains, a conformational change occurs in the β subunits and the receptor becomes an activated enzyme that is able to phosphorylate tyrosine residues on target proteins. The tyrosine kinase domains of the receptors are located on the intracellular tails of the receptor, which are part of the β chains. The activated receptor is able to autophosphorylate two tyrosine residues on the same chain as the catalytic site, and this action increases the capacity of the receptor to phosphorylate its targets. Furthermore, autophosphorylation of the receptor allows it to remain active despite dissociation of insulin from the receptor binding site. There are many intracellular targets of the insulin receptor, and these include the insulin receptor substrate (IRS) proteins, Shc, Grb, and Cbl. Stimulation of these mediators leads to activation of other pathways. The downstream effects include new gene expression and growth regulation, effects in glucose regulation, and synthesis of glycogen, lipid, and proteins. Of note, other signaling pathways also feedback to regulate the activity of the insulin receptor. For instance, phosphorylation of serine and threonine of the receptor by protein kinase A or protein kinase C decreases its tyrosine kinase activity.

Case Conclusion   GH is diagnosed with type I diabetes mellitus. She is admitted for treatment of diabetic ketoacidosis and pyelonephritis. It is felt that GH had undiagnosed type I diabetes mellitus over that last several months and that the pyelonephritis caused her to go into diabetic ketoacidosis. After a 3-day hospital stay, GH is discharged to home on an insulin regimen with close follow-up in the diabetes clinic.

Thumbnail: IGF Receptor Signaling Pathway

Phenotypes of Mouse Models with Deletion of Components of the Insulin Signaling Pathway	
Gene	**Phenotype**
Insulin receptor	Severe diabetes; postnatal death at 3 to 7 days
Insulin-like growth factor-1 (IGF-1) receptor	Growth retardation, normal glucose homeostasis
IRS-1 insulin and IGF-1 resistance	B-cell hyperplasia; metabolic syndrome
IRS-2 insulin resistance	Reduced B-cell mass; type II diabetes
IRS-3	no apparent phenotype
IRS-4	no apparent phenotype

Key Points

▶ Insulin is produced as propeptide that requires post-translational modification. First is preproinsulin, then proinsulin, and cleavage of C-peptide results in mature active insulin.

▶ Binding of insulin to its receptor results in activation of the tyrosine kinase activity intrinsic in the intracellular tail of the receptor.

▶ The insulin receptor is able to autophosphorylate its intracellular tail to augment its activity and maintain its activated state despite dissociation of its ligand.

▶ The insulin receptor acts to phosphorylate tyrosine residues on target proteins.

▶ Downstream effects of insulin signaling include gene expression, growth regulation, glucose utilization, and synthesis of glycogen, lipid, and proteins.

Questions

1. GH is discharged to home on an insulin regimen that she administers by subcutaneous injections. Which one of the following is an action of insulin?

   A. Activate catabolic processes in the muscle, liver, and adipose tissue

   B. Decrease the rate of glycogen, lipid, and protein synthesis

   C. Decrease gluconeogenesis in the liver

   D. Down-regulate cell growth and inhibit new gene expression

   E. Prevent glucose and amino acids from entering muscle and fat cells

2. A new pharmacologic agent is developed and found to activate protein kinase A activity. What effect on the insulin signaling pathway would this have?

   A. Increase autophosphorylation of the insulin receptor

   B. Inhibit the activity of the protein kinase C

   C. Decrease synthesis of glycogen

   D. Increase insulin receptor phosphorylation of tyrosine residues

   E. Decrease insulin production

HPI: KW is a previously healthy 21-year-old female college student who is brought to the hospital by her roommate. KW has difficulty giving a history but is able to indicate that she was well the previous day. She reports suddenly feeling feverish and shortly after had multiple bouts of watery diarrhea and vomiting. KW and her roommate initially attributed her symptoms to something she ate at a party the night before. However, she began to feel worse with increasing body aches, headaches, and abdominal pain. They both began worrying after noting a sunburn-like rash on KW's face and body, especially at her upper arms and legs.

PE: KW's vital signs are significant for a temperature of 38.9°C despite acetaminophen (Tylenol) taken 2 hours earlier, tachycardia to the 120s, and BP of 88/45 mm Hg, with positive orthostatics. She is obviously ill appearing with signs of dehydration. Her conjunctiva and oropharynx are erythematous. There is an impressive erythematous macular rash over her face, proximal extremities, and trunk. The cardiopulmonary exam is relatively normal except for the tachycardia, the abdomen is diffusely tender without masses, and there is no costovertebral angle tenderness. On pelvic exam, the external genitalia are normal, and on speculum exam, a soaked tampon is removed and a small amount of blood is in the vaginal vault. A CBC with differential, basic metabolic panel, LFTs, and cultures of the throat and vagina are sent.

Thought Questions

- What is toxic shock syndrome (TSS)? What is the causative agent?

- What are superantigens? How do they work?

- Describe the genetics of the T-cell receptor. How does this compare with the genetics of the immunoglobulin?

- How does antigen presentation occur?

Basic Science Review and Discussion

TSS was first described in 1978. It was diagnosed mainly in menstruating women between the ages of 12 and 24 years and was associated with the use of superabsorbent tampons. Today, the incidence of TSS in menstruating women is 6 to 7 in 100,000 annually. The disease is caused by a pyogenic toxin produced by *Staphylococcus aureus,* and colonization typically precedes disease. It has been shown that the TSS toxin (TSST) is a superantigen and is able to activate large numbers of T-cells, resulting in TSS. These symptoms can include a sudden onset of high fever (38.9°C or greater), watery diarrhea, vomiting, abdominal tenderness, myalgias, headaches, sore throat, and conjunctivitis. A erythematous, sunburn-like rash often appears on the face, proximal extremities, and trunk, with desquamation occurring within 2 weeks. Patients are ill appearing with signs of severe dehydration. The syndrome can rapidly progress to hypotensive shock within 48 hours.

Initial evaluation includes obtaining a CBC count with differentiation, electrolyte panel, BUN, creatinine, LFTs, UA, and vaginal cultures. Treatment begins with aggressive supportive therapy involving fluid and electrolyte resuscitation. With hypotensive shock, pressors are given. Many patients develop acute respiratory distress syndrome (ARDS) and are placed on mechanical ventilation. In some cases, hemodialysis is performed because of acute renal failure (ARF). Some physicians give a course of steroids to decrease the severity and duration of the illness. Antibiotic treatment, with a β-lactamase-resistant agent, is also initiated.

A 3% to 6% mortality rate is associated with TSS. The cause of death usually is due to ARDS, intractable hypotension, or hemorrhage secondary to disseminated intravascular coagulation (DIC).

T-cell Receptor Genetics To understand how superantigens work, we review TCR genetics and antigen presentation. The TCR is a transmembrane glycoprotein made up of a pair of α and β chains or γ and δ chains, and each pair is joined by a disulfide bond. Most T-cells, however, display an α-receptor and a β-receptor. Both chains of the receptor span the plasma membrane and include a short C-terminus region on the cytosolic side. The TCR resembles the immunoglobin molecule structurally, including a hypervariable sequence within the variable regions. All chains have a variable and a constant region. The TCR gene is encoded on three chromosomal regions. The genes consist of multiple variable (V), diversity (D), joining (J), and constant (C) regions. The recombination of one the various V, D, J, and C regions, the imprecision in the joining of the elements, and the different α and β or γ and δ combinations create the vast diversity in TCR in a similar manner as with immunoglobulins.

Antigen Presentation and Superantigens The cellular immune response is mediated by T-cells. T-cell activation occurs with the binding of antigenic protein fragments on the cell membranes of antigen-presenting cells (APCs) to the TCR. Foreign proteins are first internalized and digested in the lysosomes of APCs, such as by macrophages. The resulting peptides are typically less than 10 residues and are presented to the T-cell by a particular major histocompatibility complex (MHC) protein. The TCR is specific for the combination of both the MHC protein and the peptide; this is known as MHC restriction. The MHC encodes three classes of transmembrane proteins. Class I proteins present foreign peptides to cytotoxic T-cells, and the binding of this complex with the TCR leads to the secretion of perforin. Class II proteins, which are primarily seen on B-cells, macrophages, and activated T-cells, present peptides to helper T-cells. Usually, these T-cells bind with B-cells and stimulate their proliferation and differentiation. Class III proteins are components of the complement cascade. Another important part of T-cell

activation is the secretion of IL-2, a potent mitogen, responsible for T-cell proliferation.

Superantigens are molecules that can stimulate T-cells independent of an antigen-specific binding event. T-cells displaying a particular β-chain variable region (V_β) on the TCR become activated. This occurs because the superantigen is able to bind to the side of the MHC molecule and the TCR, not in the region where specific antigen binding occurs. As a consequence, multiple T-cells (not clonal) become activated, resulting in the secretion of potent cytokines. Superantigens are powerful mitogens with the ability to stimulate a biologic effect at femtomolar concentrations.

Case Conclusion   KW is admitted for presumed TSS, started on IV antibiotics, and given aggressive fluid and electrolyte resuscitation. She significantly worsens and is transferred to the ICU for ARDS, DIC, hypotensive shock requiring pressors, and ARF needing dialysis. She eventually recovers but with permanent renal impairments. The final report on the cultures obtained is positive for a penicillinase-producing *S. aureus* consistent with TSS.

Thumbnail: T-cell Receptor Pathways

It was discovered in mice that superantigens can cause clonal deletion of T-cells bearing a certain V_β chain. In these mice, entire sets of T-cells are deleted in the thymus.

Superantigens can be either an endogenous or an exogenous antigen. They do not bind in the binding site of the MHC-II molecule but directly to the MHC-II and the β chain of the TCR, then resulting in an intense proliferation response.

An example of an exogenous superantigen is the staphylococcal enterotoxin B, which has been shown to activate all TCR containing a $V_\beta 3$ or a $V_\beta 8$. An endogenous superantigen in mice is the Mls antigen, which is expressed in the thymus of mice and causes deletion (negative selection) of T-cells bearing $V_\beta 3$, $V_\beta 6$, or $V_\beta 8.1$.

Key Points

▶ TSS is caused by the *S. aureus* toxin, which is a superantigen.

▶ Superantigens act by activating all T-cells that express a specific V_β, and therefore, T-cell activation is not specific for a particular antigen.

▶ The diversity of the TCR is due to the recombination of V, D, J segments, the imprecision at the junctions, and the different α/β or γ/δ combinations.

Questions

1. A 28-year-old female presents to the ED with what appears to be a bacterial infection and sepsis. What is likely true about the immune cells in her body?

   A. In general, her T-cells become activated when TCRs recognize a peptide and an MHC protein.

   B. Her TCRs and immunoglobins both have a soluble and a membrane-bound form.

   C. Most peptides recognized by the TCRs are at least 20 amino acids in length.

   D. The diversity of her TCRs is in part due to the potential combinations among the α, β, γ, and δ chains.

   E. The superantigen causing her illness does so by inhibiting a T-cell response and cytokine secretion.

2. This patient is diagnosed with a bacterial infection associated with the production of a toxin and the toxin is suspected to be a superantigen. What part of the TCR bound by the superantigen is common in all the T-cells activated by the superantigen?

   A. V_α

   B. V_β

   C. V_δ

   D. V_γ

   E. MHC protein

3. The proteins that present peptides to T-cells were discovered because of their role in transplant rejection. Rejection occurs when tissues are transplanted between individuals with different genes in the MHC. Which of the following is true about the MHC proteins?

   A. Class I proteins consist of an α chain and a β_2-microglobulin and are involved in the complement cascade.

   B. Class II proteins are highly conserved.

   C. Class II proteins, which encode the human leukocyte antigens (HLAs), are associated with autoimmune disorders.

   D. Class II and III proteins bind peptides and are integral in antigen presentation.

   E. Class I, II, and III genes are part of the immunoglobulin gene superfamily because of the homology between themselves.

HPI: You are an intern on elective in rural Thailand working in a U.S.-sponsored clinic. AR is a 28-year-old American brought to the clinic by his co-workers. AR and his co-workers were doing field work in the rain forests for several weeks. AR is too weak, so you rely on his co-workers for a history. His co-workers report that AR started feeling ill 2 days ago and since then has had massive amounts of watery diarrhea that looks like "rice water." They also note that he has had some vomiting and complains of excruciating leg cramps. You take AR's vital signs, and he is febrile but with marked hypertension and tachycardia.

PE: AR has severe dehydration with dry mucous membranes and an absence of skin turgor. At the end of the exam, one of the co-workers says to you, "Hey, doc, is it serious? Several of us are starting to get sick with that diarrhea, too."

Thought Questions

- What is cholera? What is the pathophysiology of this disease?
- What are G-proteins and how do they work?
- What are downstream effectors of G-proteins?

Basic Science Review and Discussion

Hormones are chemical messengers that bind to cell surface receptors triggering a cascade of events within a cell. The G-protein and cAMP system is a well-studied second messenger system that functions downstream to many hormones such as epinephrine and glucagon. G-proteins serve to couple the activated hormone receptor to adenylate cyclase, the enzyme that forms cAMP from ATP. Of note, receptors that activate G-proteins share a common feature of **seven transmembrane helices.** The activation of G-proteins by these receptors is dependent not only on the binding of hormone to the receptor, but also by the phosphorylation or dephosphorylation of specific sites at the C-terminus end of the receptor.

How do G-proteins work? G-proteins are peripheral membrane proteins consisting of α, β, and γ subunits. The G-protein is always bound to either GTP (active state) or guanosine diphosphate (GDP) (inactive state) and interconvert between the two forms. The α subunit contains the GTP and GDP binding site and the GTP bound form, G_α-GTP, serves as the effector protein that activates adenylate cyclase. In the absence of hormone binding, the G-protein remains in the inactive GDP form. Once hormone binding occurs, the activated receptor triggers the release of GDP from the α subunit of the G-protein, allowing GTP to enter into the binding site. The α subunit then dissociates from the $\beta\gamma$ subunits and activates adenylate cyclase. This particular G-protein that activates adenylate cyclase is called the stimulatory G protein (G_s). **Adenylate cyclase** is also a membrane protein and converts ATP to cAMP. The downstream

effects of cAMP are many and include the activation of protein kinases. Many G_α-GTP are formed from the binding of one hormone to its receptor, resulting in the amplified response from one signaling event. G-proteins also have a built-in system of deactivation. The GTP bound to the α subunit is slowly hydrolyzed to the inactive GDP form by its own guanosine triphosphatase (GTPase) activity. The proportion of active G-proteins in a cell is dependent on the rate of exchange of GDP to GTP after a hormonal signaling event compared with the intrinsic GTPase activity of the α subunit.

Another regulator of G_s is the **inhibitory G protein** (G_i). G_i also consists of α, β, and γ subunits. Activation of G_i upon receptor stimulation leads to the dissociation of the $\beta\gamma$ subunit of G_i, and it binds to G_s, causing a reversal of adenylate cyclase activation.

This is an effective means of negative regulation because cells contain significantly more G_i than G_s.

The protein kinases that are activated by cAMP modulate target proteins by phosphorylating on serine residues in conserved sequence of Arg-Arg-X-Ser-X, where X can be any residue. One such kinase is protein kinase A, which acts downstream to the epinephrine receptor. The typical conformation of these protein kinases is that it contains two regulatory and two catalytic subunits. The regulatory subunits each contain two cAMP binding sites. In the absence of cAMP, the enzyme is inactive. However, the binding of cAMP to the two sites on each regulatory subunit causes the dissociation of the two regulatory subunits from the two catalytic subunits, which then become enzymatically active.

It is worth mentioning that there is a whole family of G-proteins that transduce different hormonal and sensory stimuli. G-proteins are known to activate **phospholipase C,** the upstream effector of the **phosphoinositide signaling cascade.** This pathway is involved in the mediation of cell secretion upon mast cell activation and chemotaxis when chemotactic receptors are bound by specific peptide. Light stimulation of rhodopsin activates the G-protein, transducin, and its downstream effect through cGMP phospho-diesterase is visual excitation. Acetylcholine (ACH) binds to the muscarinic receptor, and the associated G-protein is involved in the regulation of a potassium channel.

Pathophysiology of Cholera *Vibrio cholerae* is a "comma-shaped" **gram-negative rod** that causes cholera. It only infects humans and is transmitted by **fecal contamination** of water. The pathogenesis of cholera begins with its colonization of the small intestines, which occurs after a large number of bacteria are ingested. Approximately 1 billion organisms need to be ingested for colonization to occur because of its susceptibility to stomach acids. While in the small intestines, the organism secretes a mucinase, which dissolves the protective glycoprotein coating on intestinal cells and allows it to adhere to the intestinal cells. *V. cholerae* next secretes an endotoxin, choleragen, an 87-kd protein composed of an α subunit (α_1 peptide linked by a disulfide bond to an α_2 peptide) and five β subunits. Choleragen is able to enter the intestinal mucosal cell when its β subunits interact with the carbohydrate-rich

motifs of G_{M1} gangliosides on the enterocyte cell surface. Once within the cell, the α_1 subunit catalyzes the transfer of an ADP-ribose unit to the α subunit of G_s, which blocks the intrinsic GTPase activity of G_s and locks it into its active form. This results in a **persistently activated adenylate cyclase** in the absence of hormone stimulation. The cAMP levels become abnormally elevated, and there is excess stimulation of active transport of ions within the intestinal mucosa, ultimately leading to a large efflux of sodium ions and water into the gut.

Diagnosis of cholera during an epidemic is based on clinical judgment, and rarely, laboratory confirmation is needed. However, in diagnosis of sporadic cases, confirmation is made by obtaining a stool culture using MacConkey's agar. Treatment of cholera consists of prompt replacement of water and electrolytes. Antibiotics such as tetracycline are not needed for treatment but can shorten the duration of symptoms. With prompt hydration, fewer than 1% of patients die; otherwise, if left untreated, there is a 40% mortality rate.

Case Conclusion AR is clinically diagnosed with cholera. Although the clinic is small, it is able to run basic blood tests and the results show that he is hypokalemic, has a metabolic acidosis, and an elevated creatinine clearance. AR receives both IV and oral hydration, electrolyte replacement, and correction of his metabolic acidosis. He also receives tetracycline, which helps to shorten the course of his illness, and he is well by day 7. His co-workers were also treated and all of them recovered well.

Thumbnail: G-proteins and Adenylate Cyclase

G-proteins and their effects				
Stimulus	**Receptor**	**G protein**	**2nd messenger**	**Effect**
epinephrine	β-adrenergic receptor	G_s	adenylate cyclase	breakdown of glycogen
serotonin	serotonin receptor	G_s	adenylate cyclase	behavior and learning
acetylcholine	muscarinic receptor	G_k	potassium channel	pacemaker activity
IgE-antigen	IgE receptor	G_{plc}	phospholipase C	degranulation/secretion
light	rhodopsin	transducin	phosphodiesterase	vision pathway

Key Points

- G-proteins:
  1. Activated by receptors that share a seven-helix transmembrane motif
  2. Are composed of α, β, and γ subunits
  3. Are active when bound to GTP and inactive when bound to GDP
  4. Are activated by hormone receptor complexes leading to many active Gα-GTP formed from each bound hormone to give an amplified response
  5. Are able to deactivate by its built-in GTPase
  6. In the Gα-GTP form, activate adenylate cyclase, which leads to the formation of the second-messenger cAMP and activation of downstream protein kinases

- Cholera:
  1. Caused by the gram-negative rod *V. cholerae*
  2. Caused by a toxin, choleragen, which keeps the Gα-GTP in its active form, resulting in an efflux of sodium and water into the gut
  3. Causes massive diarrhea, which results is marked dehydration, electrolyte imbalance, and acidosis
  4. Requires immediate treatment by oral and IV hydration and electrolyte replacement

Questions

1. Epinephrine is known to bind to its receptor and cause the activation of a G-protein. The end result of this pathway is the breakdown of glycogen. Which of the following is a regulatory mechanism of this signaling pathway?
   - **A.** The phosphorylation of the C-terminus end of the G-protein, preventing the GTP-GDP exchange
   - **B.** Action of G_i by the α subunit competitively binding up available GTP
   - **C.** cAMP binding to the regulatory subunits of protein kinase A in an allosteric manner, resulting in release of the catalytic subunit
   - **D.** The intrinsic GTPase activity of the Gα to convert the active GDP form to the inactive GTP form
   - **E.** The ADP-ribosylation of G_s preventing the hydrolysis of GTP to GDP

2. A small child is brought into the ED with a hacking cough and production of copious amounts of mucus for 3 days. Her parents note a "whoop" in the cough. She is diagnosed with having pertussis, an acute tracheobronchitis caused by *Bordetella pertussis,* a gram-negative rod. *B. pertussis* produces a toxin that catalyzes the addition of ADP ribose to the G_i protein, preventing its action and thereby resulting in which of the following?
   - **A.** Inhibition of adenylate cyclase
   - **B.** Production of phosphatidylinositol 4,5-bisphosphate (PIP_2)
   - **C.** Inability of the α subunit to dissociate from $\beta\gamma$
   - **D.** Hydrolysis of GTP to GDP
   - **E..** Inhibition of phospholipase C and the phosphoinositide signaling pathway

HPI: WE is a 59-year-old man who is brought to the ED in an acute state of alcohol intoxication. He is given IV hydration and put in a stretcher to "sleep it off." Several hours later he awakes, but his nurse finds him quite confused and calls the ED resident to examine him.

PE: He is noted to have a horizontal nystagmus and ataxia that is so severe, WE has difficulty standing. After a short time, he attempts to walk and is noticed to have a wide gait. The resident notices that WE is getting just IV hydration and orders a vitamin to be added to the hydration. He also orders a neurology and psychiatry consult.

Thought Questions

- What diagnoses are WE's history and exam most consistent with?

- What vitamin did the resident most likely add to the IV?

- What are the other important vitamin deficiencies and how do they present?

Basic Science Review and Discussion

WE's symptoms are most consistent with Wernicke-Korsakoff syndrome, where Wernicke's disease describes the acute neurologic changes of the ocular nerves leading to nystagmus in this patient, as well as the ataxia, and Korsakoff's psychosis describes symptoms of drowsiness, apathy, amnesia, and confusion. This syndrome is a result of thiamine (vitamin B_1) deficiency. Vitamin deficiencies can be discussed in each system separately or collectively as a series of vitamins. Here, we present them together.

Vitamins   Vitamins are **cofactors** and **coenzymes** used throughout the body in a multitude of reactions in synthesis and maintenance of homeostasis. The key importance of vitamins is that they must primarily be obtained from our diet; they either cannot be synthesized or are not synthesized at levels necessary to meet the body's demands. Deficiencies in these vitamins can lead to various diseases. Vitamins are usually broken down into the water-soluble (the B and C) and the fat-soluble (D, E, A, and K) vitamins.

Vitamin B_1—Thiamine   Thiamine is converted to its active form, **TPP**, in the brain and liver by a specific enzyme, **thiamine diphosphotransferase.**. TPP is necessary as a cofactor for the **pyruvate dehydrogenase** and **α-ketoglutarate dehydrogenase**-catalyzed reactions, as well as the **transketolase**-catalyzed reactions of the pentose phosphate pathway. A deficiency in thiamine intake leads to a severely reduced capacity of cells to generate energy as a result of its role in these reactions.

The earliest symptoms of thiamine deficiency include constipation, appetite suppression, nausea, mental depression,

peripheral neuropathy, and fatigue. Chronic thiamine deficiency leads to more severe neurologic symptoms including ataxia, mental confusion, and loss of eye coordination (Wernicke-Korsakoff syndrome). Other clinical symptoms of prolonged thiamine deficiency are related to cardiovascular and musculature defects. Severe thiamine deficiency leads to **beriberi,** which can manifest as high cardiac output failure.

Vitamin B_2—Riboflavin   Riboflavin is the precursor for the coenzymes, **flavin mononucleotide (FMN)** and *FAD*. The enzymes that require FMN or FAD as cofactors are termed **flavoproteins.** Several flavoproteins also contain metal ions and are termed **metalloflavoproteins.** Both classes of enzymes are involved in a wide range of redox reactions, for example, **succinate dehydrogenase** and **xanthine oxidase.** During the course of the enzymatic reactions involving the flavoproteins, the reduced forms of FMN and FAD are formed, $FMNH_2$ and $FADH_2$, respectively.

Riboflavin deficiencies are rare in the United States because of the presence of adequate amounts of the vitamin in eggs, milk, meat, and cereals. Riboflavin deficiency is often seen in chronic alcoholics because of their poor dietetic habits. Symptoms associated with riboflavin deficiency include glossitis, seborrhea, angular stomatitis, cheilosis, and photophobia. Riboflavin decomposes when exposed to visible light. This characteristic can lead to riboflavin deficiencies in newborns treated for hyperbilirubinemia by phototherapy.

Vitamin B_3—Niacin   Niacin is required for the synthesis of the active forms of vitamin B_3, NAD^+ and **nicotinamide adenine dinucleotide phosphate** *($NADP^+$)*. Both NAD^+ and $NADP^+$ function as cofactors for numerous dehydrogenases, for example, lactate dehydrogenase (LDH). Both nicotinic acid and nicotinamide can serve as the dietary source of vitamin B_3. However, niacin is not a true vitamin in the strictest definition because it can be derived from the amino acid tryptophan. However, the ability to use tryptophan for niacin synthesis is inefficient (60 mg of tryptophan is required to synthesize 1 mg of niacin).

A diet deficient in niacin (as well as tryptophan) leads to glossitis of the tongue, dermatitis, weight loss, diarrhea, depression, and dementia. The severe symptoms, depression, dermatitis, and diarrhea, are associated with the condition known as **pellagra**. Several physiologic conditions and drug therapies can lead to niacin deficiency. In Hartnup disease, tryptophan absorption is impaired, and in malignant carcinoid syndrome, tryptophan metabolism is altered, resulting in excess serotonin synthesis. Isoniazid is the primary drug for the treatment of tuberculosis.

Interestingly, nicotinic acid (but not nicotinamide) when administered in pharmacologic doses of 2–4 g/day lowers plasma cholesterol levels and has been shown to be a useful therapeutic for hypercholesterolemia. The major action of nicotinic acid in this capacity is a reduction in fatty acid mobilization from adipose tissue. Although nicotinic acid therapy lowers blood cholesterol levels, it also causes a depletion of glycogen stores and fat reserves in skeletal and cardiac muscle. Additionally, there is an elevation in blood glucose level and uric acid production. For these reasons, nicotinic acid therapy is not recommended for diabetics or persons who suffer from gout.

Vitamin B$_5$—Pantothenic Acid Pantothenic acid is formed from β-alanine and pantoic acid. Pantothenate is required for synthesis of **CoA** (Figure 20-1) and is a component of the ACP domain of fatty acid synthase. Thus, pantothenate is required for the metabolism of carbohydrate via the TCA cycle and all fats and proteins. At least 70 enzymes have been identified as requiring CoA or ACP derivatives for their function.

Deficiency of pantothenic acid is extremely rare because of its widespread distribution in whole-grain cereals, legumes, and meat. Symptoms of pantothenate deficiency are diffi-

cult to assess because they are subtle and resemble those of other B vitamin deficiencies.

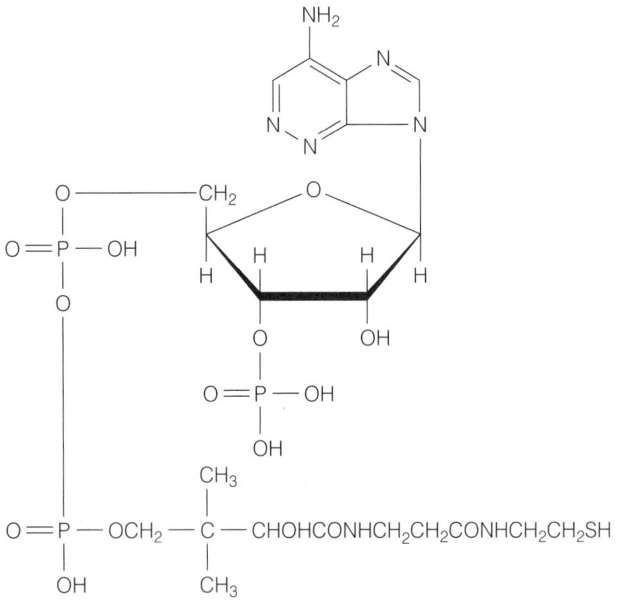

Vitamin B$_6$—Pyridoxine **Pyridoxal, pyridoxamine,** and **pyridoxine** are collectively known as **vitamin B$_6$**. All three compounds are efficiently converted to the biologically active form of vitamin B$_6$, **pyridoxal phosphate** (PLP), catalyzed by the ATP-requiring enzyme **pyridoxal kinase.** PLP functions as a cofactor in enzymes involved in transamination reactions required for the synthesis and catabolism of the amino acids, as well as in glycogenolysis as a cofactor for **glycogen phosphorylase.** Deficiencies of vitamin B$_6$ are rare and usually are related to an overall deficiency of all the B-complex vitamins. Isoniazid and penicillamine are drugs that complex with pyridoxal and PLP, resulting in a deficiency in this vitamin.

Vitamin B$_{12}$—Cobalamin Vitamin B$_{12}$ is composed of a complex tetrapyrrol ring structure (corrin ring) and a cobalt ion in the center. It is synthesized exclusively by microorganisms and is found in the liver of animals bound to protein as methylcobalamin or 5'-deoxyadenosylcobalamin. The vitamin must be hydrolyzed from protein in order to be active. Hydrolysis occurs in the stomach by gastric acids or the intestines by trypsin digestion following consumption of animal meat. The vitamin is then bound by **intrinsic factor** (IF), a protein secreted by parietal cells of the stomach, and carried to the ileum where it is absorbed. Following absorption, the vitamin is transported to the liver in the blood bound to **transcobalamin II** (TCII).

Only two clinically significant reactions in the body require vitamin B$_{12}$ as a cofactor. During the catabolism of fatty acids with an odd number of carbon atoms and the amino acids valine, isoleucine, and threonine, the resultant propionyl-CoA is converted to succinyl-CoA for oxidation in the TCA cycle. One of the enzymes in this pathway, **methylmalonyl-CoA mutase**, requires vitamin B$_{12}$ as a cofactor in the conversion of methylmalonyl-CoA to succinyl-CoA. The 5'-deoxyadenosine derivative of cobalamin is required for this reaction. The second reaction requiring vitamin B$_{12}$ catalyzes the conversion of homocysteine to methionine and is catalyzed by **methionine synthase.** This reaction results in the transfer of the methyl group from N^5-methyl-tetrahydrofolate to hydroxocobalamin generating THF and methylcobalamin during the process of the conversion.

The liver can store up to 6 years' worth of vitamin B$_{12}$, so deficiencies in this vitamin are rare. Pernicious anemia is a megaloblastic anemia resulting from vitamin B$_{12}$ deficiency that develops as a result of a lack of IF in the stomach leading to malabsorption of the vitamin. The anemia results from impaired DNA synthesis caused by a block in purine and thymidine biosynthesis. The block in nucleotide biosynthesis is a consequence of the effect of vitamin B$_{12}$ on folate metabolism. When vitamin B$_{12}$ is deficient, essentially all of the folate becomes trapped as the N^5-methyltetrahy-

Figure 20-1 The molecular structure of CoA.

drofolate derivative as a result of the loss of functional *methionine synthase.* This trapping prevents the synthesis of other THF derivatives required for the purine and thymidine nucleotide biosynthesis pathways.

Neurologic complications also are associated with vitamin B_{12} deficiency and result from a progressive demyelination of nerve cells. The demyelination is thought to result from the increase in methylmalonyl-CoA that results from vitamin B_{12} deficiency. Methylmalonyl-CoA is a competitive inhibitor of malonyl-CoA in fatty acid biosynthesis, as well as being able to substitute for malonyl-CoA in any fatty acid biosynthesis that may occur. Because the myelin sheath is in continual flux, the methylmalonyl-CoA-induced inhibition of fatty acid synthesis results in the eventual destruction of the sheath.

Folic Acid   Folic acid is a conjugated molecule consisting of a pteridine ring structure linked to *p*-aminobenzoic acid **(PABA)** that forms pteroic acid. Folic acid itself is then generated through the conjugation of glutamic acid residues to pteroic acid. Folic acid is obtained primarily from yeasts and leafy vegetables, as well as animal liver. Animals cannot synthesize PABA and cannot attach glutamate residues to pteroic acid, so they require folate intake in the diet.

When stored in the liver or ingested, folic acid exists in a polyglutamate form. Intestinal mucosal cells remove some of the glutamate residues through the action of the lysosomal enzyme **conjugase.** The removal of glutamate residues makes folate less negatively charged (from the polyglutamic acids) and therefore more capable of passing through the basal laminal membrane of the epithelial cells of the intestine and into the bloodstream. Folic acid (Figure 20-2) is reduced primarily within liver cells, where it is also stored to THF through the action of **DHFR,** an NADPH-requiring enzyme. The function of THF derivatives is to carry and transfer various forms of one-carbon units during biosynthetic reactions. The one-carbon units are either methyl, methylene, methenyl, formyl, or formimino groups.

Folate deficiency results in complications nearly identical to those described for vitamin B_{12} deficiency. The most pronounced effect of folate deficiency on cellular processes is

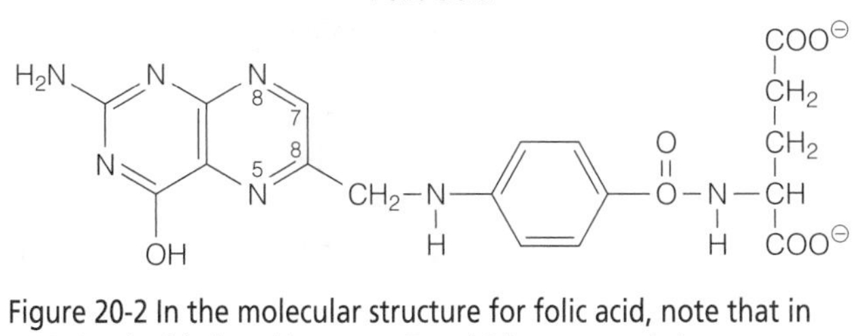

on DNA synthesis. This is due to an impairment in dTMP synthesis, which leads to cell cycle arrest in the S phase of rapidly proliferating cells, in particular hematopoietic cells. The result is **megaloblastic anemia** similar to vitamin B_{12} deficiency. The inability to synthesize DNA during erythrocyte maturation leads to abnormally large erythrocytes termed **macrocytic anemia.**

Folate deficiencies are rare because of the adequate presence of folate in food. Poor dietary habits can lead to folate deficiency. The predominant causes of folate deficiency in nonalcoholics include impaired absorption or metabolism or an increased demand for the vitamin. The predominant condition requiring an increase in the daily intake of folate is pregnancy. Folate deficiency has been associated with fetal anomalies such as spina bifida, and its supplementation has been shown to decrease these defects. Certain drugs such as anticonvulsants and oral contraceptives can impair the absorption of folate. Anticonvulsants also increase the rate of folate metabolism.

Biotin   Biotin is the cofactor required of enzymes that are involved in carboxylation reactions **(acetyl-CoA carboxylase and pyruvate carboxylase).** Biotin is found in numerous foods and is synthesized by intestinal bacteria, and as such, deficiencies of the vitamin are rare. Deficiencies are generally seen only after long antibiotic therapies that deplete the intestinal fauna or after excessive consumption of raw eggs. The latter is due to the affinity of the egg-white protein, **avidin,** for biotin preventing intestinal absorption of the biotin.

Vitamin C—Ascorbic Acid   Ascorbic acid is derived from glucose via the uronic acid pathway. The enzyme L-gulonolactone oxidase, which is responsible for the conversion of gulonolactone to ascorbic acid, is absent in primates, making ascorbic acid required in the diet. The active form of vitamin C is ascorbate acid itself. The main function of ascorbate is to act as a reducing agent in a number of different reactions. Vitamin C has the potential to reduce cytochromes *a* and *c* of the respiratory chain, as well as molecular oxygen. The most important reaction requiring ascorbate as a cofactor is the hydroxylation of proline residues in collagen. Vitamin C is, therefore, required for the maintenance of normal connective tissue and for wound healing because synthesis of connective tissue is the first event in wound tissue remodeling. Vitamin C also is necessary for bone remodeling because of the presence of collagen in the organic matrix of bones.

Deficiency in vitamin C leads to the disease **scurvy,** because of its role in the post-translational modification of collagens. Scurvy is characterized by easily bruised skin, muscle fatigue, soft swollen gums, decreased wound healing and hemorrhaging, osteoporosis, and anemia. Vitamin C is readily absorbed, so the primary cause of vitamin C deficiency is poor diet and/or an increased requirement. The

Folic acid

Figure 20-2 In the molecular structure for folic acid, note that in DHF the double bond between 7 and 8 is gone, and these atoms are bound to hydrogen molecules. In THF, the same is true for 5 and 6 as well.

primary physiologic state leading to an increased requirement for vitamin C is severe stress (or trauma). This is due to a rapid depletion in the adrenal stores of the vitamin. The reason for the decrease in adrenal vitamin C levels is unclear but may be due either to redistribution of the vitamin to areas that need it or to an overall increased utilization.

Vitamin A   Vitamin A consists of three biologically active molecules, **retinol, retinal** (retinaldehyde), and **retinoic acid.** Each of these compounds is derived from the plant precursor molecule, **β-carotene** (a member of a family of molecules known as **carotenoids**). β-Carotene, which consists of two molecules of retinal linked at their aldehyde ends, is also referred to as the provitamin form of vitamin A.

Photoreception in the eye is the function of two specialized cell types located in the retina: the rod and the cone cells. Both rod and cone cells contain a photoreceptor pigment in their membranes. The photosensitive compound of most mammalian eyes is a protein called **opsin,** to which is covalently coupled an aldehyde of vitamin A. The opsin of rod cells is called **scotopsin.** The photoreceptor of rod cells is specifically called **rhodopsin,** or **visual purple.** This compound is a complex between scotopsin and the 11-*cis*-retinal (also called 11-*cis*-retinene) form of vitamin A.

Vitamin A is stored in the liver, and deficiency of the vitamin occurs only after prolonged lack of dietary intake. The earliest symptom of vitamin A deficiency is **night blindness.** Additional early symptoms include follicular hyperkeratosis, increased susceptibility to infection and cancer and anemia equivalent to iron-deficient anemia. Prolonged lack of vitamin A leads to deterioration of the eye tissue through progressive keratinization of the cornea, a condition known as **xerophthalmia.** The increased risk of cancer in vitamin deficiency is thought to be the result of a depletion in β-carotene, which is a very effective antioxidant and is suspected to reduce the risk of cancers known to be initiated by the production of free radicals. Of particular interest is the potential benefit of increased β-carotene intake to reduce the risk of lung cancer in smokers. However, caution needs to be taken when increasing the intake of any of the lipid-soluble vitamins. Excess accumulation of vitamin A in the liver can lead to toxicity, which manifests as bone pain, hepatosplenomegaly, nausea, and diarrhea.

Vitamin D   Vitamin D is a steroid hormone that functions to regulate specific gene expression following interaction with its intracellular receptor. The biologically active form of the hormone is 1,25-dihydroxyvitamin D_3 (1,25-[OH]$_2D_3$, also termed **calcitriol**). Calcitriol functions primarily to regulate calcium and phosphorous homeostasis.

Active calcitriol is derived from **ergosterol** (produced in plants) and from **7-dehydrocholesterol** (produced in the skin). **Ergocalciferol** (vitamin D_2) is formed by ultraviolet (UV) irradiation of ergosterol. In the skin 7-dehydrocholes-terol is converted to **cholecalciferol** (vitamin D_3) following UV irradiation. Vitamin D_2 and D_3 are processed to D_2-calcitriol and D_3-calcitriol, respectively, by the same enzymatic pathways in the body. Cholecalciferol is absorbed from the intestine and transported to the liver bound to a specific **vitamin D-binding protein.** In the liver, cholecalciferol is hydroxylated at the 25 position by a specific D_3-25-hydroxylase, generating 25-hydroxyvitamin D_3 (25-[OH]D_3), which is the major circulating form of vitamin D. Conversion of 25-hydroxyvitamin D_3 to its biologically active form, calcitriol, occurs through the activity of a specific D_3-1-hydroxylase present in the proximal convoluted tubules of the kidneys, as well as in bone and placenta. 25-Hydroxyvitamin D_3 can also be hydroxylated at the 24 position by a specific D_3-24-hydroxylase in the kidneys, intestine, placenta, and cartilage.

Calcitriol functions in concert with **parathyroid hormone (PTH)** and **calcitonin** to regulate serum calcium and phosphorous levels. PTH is released in response to low serum calcium levels and induces the production of calcitriol. In contrast, reduced levels of PTH stimulate synthesis of the inactive 24,25-(OH)$_2D_3$. In the intestinal epithelium, calcitriol functions as a steroid hormone in inducing the expression of calbindinD$_{28K}$, a protein involved in intestinal calcium absorption. The increased absorption of calcium ions requires concomitant absorption of a negatively charged counter ion to maintain electrical neutrality. The predominant counter ion is P_i. When plasma calcium levels fall, the major sites of action of calcitriol and PTH are bone, where they stimulate bone resorption, and the kidneys, where they inhibit calcium excretion by stimulating reabsorption by the distal tubules.

The role of calcitonin in calcium homeostasis is to decrease elevated serum calcium levels by inhibiting bone resorption. As a result of the addition of vitamin D to milk, deficiencies in this vitamin are rare in this country. The main symptom of vitamin D deficiency in children is **rickets** and in adults is **osteomalacia.** Rickets is characterized by improper mineralization during the development of the bones, resulting in soft bones. Osteomalacia is characterized by demineralization of previously formed bone, leading to increased softness and susceptibility to fracture.

Vitamin E   Vitamin E is a mixture of several related compounds known as **tocopherols.** The α-tocopherol molecule is the most potent of the tocopherols. Vitamin E is absorbed from the intestines packaged in chylomicrons. It is delivered to the tissues via chylomicron transport and then to the liver through chylomicron remnant uptake. The liver can export vitamin E in VLDLs. Because of its lipophilic nature, vitamin E accumulates in cellular membranes, fat deposits, and other circulating lipoproteins. The major site of vitamin E storage is in adipose tissue.

The major function of vitamin E is to act as a natural **antioxidant** by scavenging free radicals and molecular oxygen. In particular, vitamin E is important for preventing peroxidation of polyunsaturated membrane fatty acids. The vitamins E and C are inter-related in their antioxidant capabilities. Active α-tocopherol can be regenerated by interaction with vitamin C following scavenge of a peroxy-free radical. Alternatively, α-tocopherol can scavenge two peroxy-free radicals and then be conjugated to glucuronate for excretion in the bile.

No major disease states have been found to be associated with vitamin E deficiency, because of adequate levels in the average U.S. diet. The major symptom of vitamin E deficiency in humans is an increase in RBC fragility. Because vitamin E is absorbed from the intestines in chylomicrons, any fat malabsorption diseases can lead to deficiencies in vitamin E intake. Neurologic disorders have been associated with vitamin E deficiencies associated with fat malabsorptive disorders. Increased intake of vitamin E is recommended in premature infants who are fed formulas that are low in the vitamin as well as in persons consuming a diet high in polyunsaturated fatty acids. Polyunsaturated fatty acids tend to form free radicals on exposure to oxygen, which may lead to an increased risk of certain cancers.

Vitamin K The K vitamins exist naturally as K_1 (phytylmenaquinone) in green vegetables, K_2 (multiprenylmenaquinone) in intestinal bacteria, and K_3 in synthetic menadione. The major function of the K vitamins is in the maintenance of normal levels of the blood-clotting proteins, factors II, VII, IX, X, and protein C and protein S, which are synthesized in the liver as inactive precursor proteins. Conversion from inactive to active clotting factor requires a post-translational modification of specific glutamate (E) residues. This modification is a carboxylation reaction, and the enzyme responsible requires vitamin K as a cofactor. During the carboxylation reaction, a reduced hydroquinone form of vitamin K is converted to a 2,3-epoxide form. The regeneration of the hydroquinone form requires an uncharacterized reductase. This latter reaction is the site of action of the dicumarol-based anticoagulants such as **warfarin**.

Naturally occurring vitamin K is absorbed from the intestines only in the presence of bile salts and other lipids through interaction with chylomicrons. Therefore, fat malabsorptive diseases can result in vitamin K deficiency. The synthetic vitamin K_3 is water soluble and absorbed irrespective of the presence of intestinal lipids and bile. Because the vitamin K_2 form is synthesized by intestinal bacteria, deficiency of the vitamin in adults is rare. However, long-term antibiotic treatment can lead to deficiency in adults. The intestine of newborn infants is sterile, so vitamin K deficiency in infants is possible if lacking from the early diet.

Case Conclusion The resident added 100 mg of thiamine to WE's IV infusion, and he was admitted to the hospital, where he receive daily intramuscular (IM) injections of thiamine. He also received folate and vitamin B_{12} supplementation when it was noted that he had a macrocytic anemia. His acute symptoms slowly resolved over the ensuing 3 to 4 days, and concerned about these symptoms, he vowed never to take another drink.

Thumbnail: Vitamin Function

Vitamin Deficiencies

Vitamin deficiency	Disease caused
Vitamin B_1 (thiamine)	Wernicke-Korsakoff syndrome; beriberi
Vitamin B_2 (riboflavin)	Glossitis, stomatitis, cheilosis, photophobia
Vitamin B_3 (niacin)	Pellagra (depression, dermatitis, diarrhea); also glossitis, weight loss, dementia
Vitamin B_5 (pantothenic acid)	Rare, findings are subtle, similar to other B vitamin deficiencies
Vitamin B_6 (pyridoxine)	Rare, findings are subtle, similar to other B vitamin deficiencies
Vitamin B_{12} (cobalamin)	Pernicious anemia, neurologic disease related to progressive demyelination
Folic acid	Macrocytic anemia, similar to B_{12}
Biotin	Rare
Vitamin C (ascorbic acid)	Scurvy
Vitamin A	Night blindness, xerophthalmia
Vitamin D	Rickets, osteomalacia
Vitamin E	Hemolysis, neurologic disorders
Vitamin K	Coagulopathy, bleeding disorder

Key Points

- Vitamins are **cofactors** and **coenzymes** used throughout the body in a multitude of reactions in synthesis and maintenance of homeostasis.
- The key importance of vitamins is that they must primarily be obtained from our diet.
- While some vitamins are synthesized by the body, it is not at adequate levels.
- Deficiencies in vitamins can lead to various diseases shown in the thumbnail.

Questions

1. A 46-year-old man presents with progressive fatigue and weakness. He notices tingling in his lower extremities but attributes these symptoms to his being on his feet all the time as a manager of a local pizza restaurant. On neurologic exam, he actually has decreased position sense and vibration sense. His hematocrit is 28, with an elevated mean corpuscular volume (MCV) of 114. His disease can most likely be attributed to a deficiency in which vitamin?

   A. Vitamin A
   B. Vitamin B_{12}
   C. Vitamin C
   D. Vitamin D
   E. Vitamin E
   F. Vitamin K
   G. Biotin

2. Another employee at the same restaurant presents after he notices that a bruise he received 3 weeks ago is not resolving. He also has a burn from an oven from 6 weeks ago, which is still slowly healing. On exam, he has swollen gums, and a bone density measurement shows osteoporosis. His disease can most likely be attributed to a deficiency in which vitamin?

   A. Vitamin A
   B. Vitamin B_{12}
   C. Vitamin C
   D. Vitamin D
   E. Vitamin E
   F. Vitamin K
   G. Biotin

Answer Key—Part I: Biochemistry

Case 1
1 E
2 D

Case 2
1 D
2 D

Case 3
1 B
2 A
3 B

Case 4
1 B
2 E
3 C

Case 5
1 D
2 A
3 E

Case 6
1 C
2 A
3 B

Case 7
1 E
2 C

Case 8
1 A
2 C

Case 9
1 A
2 B

Case 10
1 D
2 C

Case 11
1 A
2 A
3 E

Case 12
1 B
2 D
3 C

Case 13
1 C
2 C
3 D

Case 14
1 D
2 D
3 A
4 A

Case 15
1 B
2 D

Case 16
1 A
2 C

Case 17
1 C
2 C

Case 18
1 A
2 B
3 C

Case 19
1 C
2 C

Case 20
1 B
2 C

Part II

Genetics

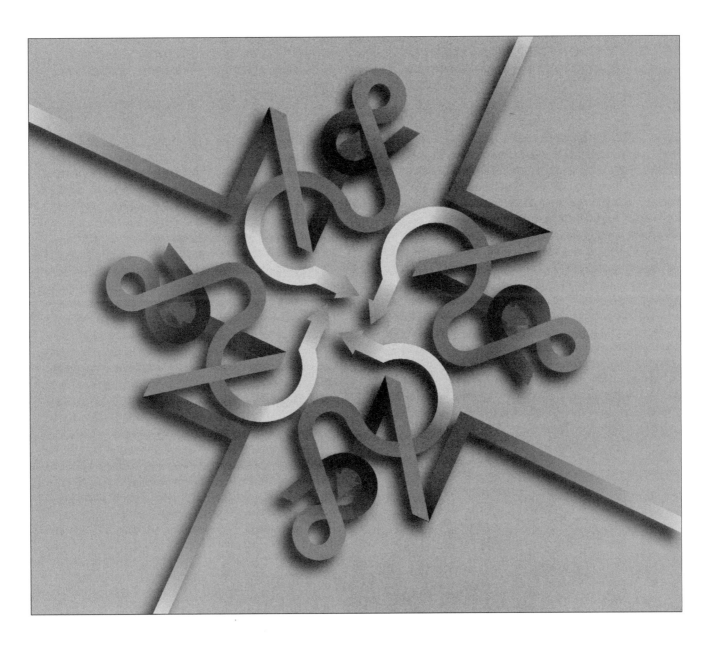

> **HPI:** A 19-year-old man comes to your office with a complaint of "droopy eyelids." He notes a 2-year history of intermittent facial weakness and over the past 6 months has had increasing difficulty keeping his eyes open. He has been otherwise healthy and denies any past diseases. The patient's family history is significant for a grandmother with cardiac arrhythmias, who died suddenly at the age of 65 years. His father and an aunt both developed cataracts and mild hand weakness in their 40s. He also has a 16-year-old cousin with multiple illnesses including neck and extremity weakness, chronic GI tract obstruction, and intellectual impairment.
>
> **PE:** The patient is a thin-appearing man with limited facial expressions. He has a narrow face and on neurologic exam has ptosis and mildly slurred speech. The remainder of his exam is normal.
>
> **Labs:** A creatine kinase level is mildly elevated at 250 U/L (normal < 200 U/L). A muscle biopsy shows mild muscle fiber atrophy and other nonspecific myopathic changes. DNA analysis shows that the patient has approximately 200 CTG repeats present in a protein kinase gene on chromosome 19. (See case pedigree in Figure 21-1.)

Thought Questions

- What is the most likely diagnosis?

- What is the inheritance pattern of this disease?

- What is the significance of the DNA analysis results?

- How would you counsel the patient on the risk to future children?

Basic Science Review and Discussion

Syndrome Description **Myotonic dystrophy** is an **autosomal dominant (AD)** disorder and the most common muscular dystrophy, with an incidence of 1 in 8000. The disease is slowly progressive and involves multiple organ systems including skeletal, cardiac, GI, and respiratory systems. The onset of symptoms is usually after puberty with characteristic manifestations of **muscle weakness,** especially of the face and extremities, with progressive involvement of the proximal muscles. Smooth muscle involvement can lead to cardiac arrhythmias, decreased GI tract motility, and respiratory dysfunction. **Myotonia** is the inability to relax voluntary muscles after contraction. The most noticeable symptom may be an inability to relax the hand after a grip, but symptoms are generally not severe enough to require treatment. Other associated symptoms of myotonic dystrophy include cataracts, testicular atrophy, and mental retardation.

Muscle biopsy reveals fiber atrophy, although serum creatine kinase level is usually normal or only mildly elevated. A definitive diagnosis can be made by DNA analysis with either PCR or Southern blot analysis to determine the number of trinucleotide repeats present in the myotonic dystrophy gene. There is no specific treatment for myotonic dystrophy. Ankle supports or leg braces can help with distal weakness, pacemakers can be used for cardiomyopathy, and cataracts can be surgically removed.

Autosomal Dominant Inheritance The myotonic dystrophy gene is located on chromosome 19 and encodes for a protein kinase. It is inherited in an AD pattern and has several distinguishing characteristics. AD diseases affect an **equal proportion of men and women.** Because every carrier of the mutation is affected, the pedigree shows **no skipped generations.** Finally, unlike X-linked or mitochondrial diseases, **fathers can pass the mutation to their sons.** The most common pairing is between an affected heterozygote and a normal individual. Half of their offspring will be normal, whereas the other half will be symptomatic carriers. Other common AD disorders include Huntington's disease, neurofibromatosis type 1, familial hypercholesterolemia, and postaxial polydactyly (extra fingers or toes).

Anticipation and Repeat Expansion The genetic cause of myotonic dystrophy is an expanding CTG trinucleotide repeat within a protein kinase gene on chromosome 19. An interesting phenomenon in familial myotonic dystrophy is that later generations afflicted with the mutation frequently have an earlier age at onset and more severe disease. This concept is termed **anticipation** and is caused by

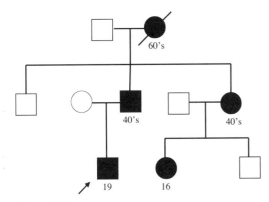

Figure 21-1

the increasing number of trinucleotide repeats found in the myotonic dystrophy gene in successive generations. Normal individuals have between 5 and 30 copies of the repeat, whereas affected individuals have more than 50 and patients with severe cases can have hundreds or thousands of copies of the CTG repeat within the gene. Other disorders caused by such trinucleotide repeat expansions include Huntington's disease (CAG), spinal and bulbar muscular atrophy (CAG), fragile X syndrome (CGG), and Friedreich's ataxia (GAA).

Case Conclusion   The patient is started on annual cardiac exams with ECGs and counseled on his increased risk of eventual cardiac, pulmonary, and GI complications. The patient's cousin is also tested for trinucleotide expansions and is found to have more than 1000 copies of the CTG repeat.

Thumbnail: Autosomal Dominant Inheritance

Diseases Associated with Trinucleotide Repeat Expansions		
Disease	**Repeat**	**Description**
Myotonic dystrophy	CTG	Facial/extremity weakness, cardiomyopathy, GI tract obstruction, respiratory tract muscle weakness, cataracts, testicular atrophy, and mental retardation
Fragile X syndrome	CGG	Mental retardation, macro-orchism in men, large ears, prominent jaw
Friedreich's ataxia	GAA	Cerebellar dysfunction, limb ataxia, sensory defects, cardiomyopathy
Huntington's disease	CAG	Loss of motor control (chorea), dementia
Spinal and bulbar muscular atrophy	CAG	Lower motor neuron disease, androgen insensitivity

Key Points

▶ Myotonic dystrophy is an AD disorder.
▶ AD disorders have the following characteristics:
  1. Affects men and women equally
  2. Does not skip generations
  3. Fathers can transmit disease to sons

▶ Anticipation defines the earlier onset and increasing severity of a disease from one generation to the next. In the presented case, this is caused by an expanding trinucleotide repeat in a gene on chromosome 19.

Questions

1. The patient meets a woman at a myotonic dystrophy support group who is also affected by the disease. They decide to marry but are very concerned about passing the disorder to their offspring. If they eventually have two children, what is the chance that neither child will inherit the chromosomal abnormality?

   A. 50%
   B. 33.3%
   C. 25%
   D. 6.25%
   E. 0%

2. Myotonic dystrophy is inherited in an AD fashion. The AD trait can share similar characteristics with the pedigree of other inheritance patterns (e.g., AR and sex linked). Which of the following is true about the inheritance pattern of both AD and X-linked dominant disorders?

   A. Men and women are affected in equal proportions.
   B. Affected women have a 50% chance of passing the diseased allele to their children.
   C. Fathers cannot pass the mutation to their sons.
   D. Skipped generations are commonly seen.
   E. Men have a 100% chance of passing the mutation to their daughters.

3. A 35-year-old woman presents to your office with a complaint of abnormal, jerky facial and body movements. Over the past few years, her memory has deteriorated and she is becoming more depressed. The patient denies any significant family history but states that her father committed suicide when he was 40 years of age. Which of the following statements is true about the likely diagnosis?

   A. It is caused by a CTG trinucleotide repeat expansion.
   B. It is inherited in a sex-linked pattern.
   C. It is inherited in an AD pattern.
   D. Anticipation is not a factor in disease transmission.
   E. Dementia is not a common feature of this disease.

4. Molecular genetic techniques are becoming the standard methods for the diagnosis of many genetic disorders. Which technique is described by the following protocol: electrophoresis of DNA fragments through a gel, transfer to a membrane, hybridize with a labeled probe, and expose to x-ray film?

   A. PCR
   B. Western blot analysis
   C. Southern blot analysis
   D. Fluorescence in situ hybridization (FISH)
   E. Northern blot analysis

HPI: FC is a 5-year-old boy with failure to thrive and chronic lung disease. Since age 11 months, he has suffered from malabsorption with increased fat content in the stools. In addition, he has recurrent, chronic bacterial lung infections often requiring hospitalization. Two weeks ago, he had an exacerbation of his cough and wheezing requiring hospitalization. Chest x-ray was consistent with bilateral lobar pneumonia. He was treated with systemic broad-spectrum antibiotics and intensive respiratory therapy. *Staphylococcus aureus* was isolated from his sputum. His medical history is significant for intestinal obstruction as a neonate. His parents are of Irish and German ancestry and are related only by marriage. He has an older sister who is healthy. No other family member is affected by a similar condition on either side of the family (Figure 22-1). Although a tentative diagnosis has been raised in the past, the parents have come to you to try to establish a definitive diagnosis and for genetic counseling.

Thought Questions

- What is the most likely diagnosis? How would you confirm it?

- What is the natural history and life expectancy of this disease?

- What treatment strategies are recommended for these patients?

- Which inheritance pattern does this pedigree suggest?

Basic Science Review and Discussion

Cystic Fibrosis   The association of symptoms presented is highly suggestive of cystic fibrosis (CF). The classically clinical triad consist of (1) chronic pulmonary obstruction and infections, (2) exocrine pancreatic insufficiency, and (3) elevations of both chloride and sodium concentration in sweat. It is the most common autosomal recessive (AR) disease in white populations, affecting about 1 in every 2500 to 3000 newborns.

In a patient with clinical suspicion of CF, a chloride sweat test result of more than 60 mmol/L confirms the diagnosis. Immunoreactive trypsin has been used as a screening test in

newborns but requires a confirmatory test because of its poor specificity. DNA testing is helpful in confirming the diagnosis in atypical cases and is essential for prenatal diagnosis.

Natural History   Sixty percent of patients with CF are diagnosed before 1 year and 90% by 10 years of age. Eighty-five percent of patients have pancreatic insufficiency manifested by chronic malabsorption and failure to thrive. Almost all patients with CF have chronic lung disease resulting from recurrent infections, leading eventually to irreversible lung damage and strain on the right ventricle (cor pulmonale). Nearly all of male individuals with CF are infertile because of the absence of the vas deferens. Chronic lung disease and its sequelae are the life-limiting factor for most patients with CF. Survival is currently 30 years for patients with CF in the United States.

Management strategies consist of improving nutritional status, preservation of lung function, decreasing the rate and treating complications, and ensuring psychosocial well-being. Exocrine pancreatic insufficiency can be effectively treated with enzyme replacement. Lung conservation is achieved by facilitating clearance of mucus and control of infection. Gene therapy is still investigational.

Inheritance   The family tree shown is not characteristic of any particular inheritance pattern but is commonly seen in AR disorders. There are three features that suggest AR inheritance: It affects both men and women in equal proportions; it typically affects individuals in one generation of a single sibship; and it does not occur in prior or subsequent generations. Consanguinity is more frequently seen in families with AR traits than in the general population. Recessive traits require that the mutant allele is present in a double dose (homozygosity), although for most AR disorders, affected individuals have two allelic mutations at the same locus (compound heterozygote, e.g., ΔF508/G542X, two of the most common mutations in CF).

Prenatal Diagnosis   CF is one of a handful of diseases that are now commonly screened for via prenatal diagnosis. In

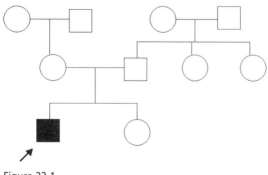

Figure 22-1

the case of screening for AR disorders like CF, usually the mother is screened first. If her test returns negative, then screening often stops there because the child can be at worst, a carrier. If her screen returns positive, then the father is screened. If his screen returns negative, again the child can at worst be a carrier. If he is positive as well, then the fetus has a 25% chance of being affected, and invasive confirmatory testing is offered via either CVS or amniocentesis to obtain fetal cells. If the fetus is homozygous recessive, termination of the pregnancy may be an option for some couples because there is no effective treatment for this devastating condition. Because the prenatal diagnostic procedures are not benign, patients need to weigh the decision regarding these options carefully after thorough counseling. In the case of CF screening, the parental screening can be further complicated, because not all of the mutations in the CF gene are identified, so the detection rate is not 100%. Despite these limitations, CF screening is offered to any pregnant woman or couple considering pregnancy in the United States.

Case Conclusion   FC undergoes DNA testing and is found to be homozygous for the △F508 mutation. Commercially available DNA tests typically screen between 12 and 72 of the most common CF mutations, with a sensitivity up to 97% for Ashkenazi Jews and more than 92% of northern Europeans, but as low as 60% in other populations. The cystic fibrosis transmembrane regulator (CFTR) genotype has a strong correlation with the phenotype in terms of age at disease onset, pancreatic insufficiency, and sweat chloride content. The correlation with pulmonary disease is less clear.

Thumbnail: Autosomal Recessive Inheritance

CF is the most common AR disorder in whites (1/3000 newborns)

Carrier frequency in whites is 1 in 30.

Diagnosis: Elevated chloride level in sweat glands; DNA analysis in cases of equivocal results

Symptoms: Exocrine pancreatic insufficiency, recurrent pulmonary infections

Infertility in men, secondary to absence of vas deferens

Normal intelligence, decreased survival (mean, 30 years)

Genetics: More than 400 mutations known; △F508 the most common

CFTR gene chromosome 7q31, gene product CFTR protein

Mutations cause alterations in chloride transport and mucin secretion

Higher frequency of carriers than expected likely explained by *heterozygote advantage*

Key Points

▶ AR disorders manifest only when the mutant allele is present in double dose.

▶ Most AR diseases occur as a result of two different mutations at the same locus (compound heterozygotes).

▶ Parents of children with traits are obligate heterozygotes or carriers and are not affected.

▶ Higher incidence of consanguinity in AR disorders.

Questions

1. The underlying mechanism responsible for CF is which of the following?
   A. Defect in cholesterol synthesis
   B. Chloride channel abnormality
   C. Autoimmune response
   D. Calcium channel defect
   E. None of the above

2. A few years later FC's older sister is considering pregnancy. Her husband is of northern European ancestry. Assuming a carrier frequency of 1 in 25 for northern Europeans, their chances of having an affected child with the same condition as her brother is what?
   A. 1 in 200
   B. 1 in 150
   C. 1 in 100
   D. 1 in 75
   E. 1 in 4

3. The couple decides to undergo carrier screening for 72 of the most common mutations of this disorder. She is a carrier of one of the mutations screened. The husband screens negative for all of the 72 mutations tested. They decide to get pregnant. However, an ultrasound of the fetus revealed "echogenic bowel," the sonographic correlate of meconium ileus. This can be explained by what?
   A. Nonpaternity
   B. Affected heterozygote
   C. Father of fetus is carrier of mutation not identified by panel used
   D. A and C are correct
   E. A, B, and C are correct

HPI: WL is a 4-year-old boy who is brought to your office by his parents for a routine pediatric checkup. His mother states that he has always been a very active child, but that over the past year, he has become clumsier, is falling more frequently, and has a hard time getting up from a sitting or lying position. He has also been increasingly tired while climbing the stairs to their family's third-floor floor apartment and now needs to rest several times along the way. WL has had no significant medical problems and so far has reached all of his developmental milestones. His mother adds that her older brother was disabled for much of his life and had died in his late teens of a respiratory tract infection. She has two healthy parents and a sister with a 1-year-old son who is reportedly normal (Figure 23-1).

PE: WL has mild spine lordosis, proximal muscle weakness, enlargement of the bilateral calf muscles, and slight contractures of the Achilles tendon. He has a positive Gowers sign (using his arms to push up the body and to climb up the thighs when rising from a sitting position) and a waddling gait when walking. The remainder of his exam is normal.

Labs: Creatine kinase level is grossly elevated, at 3000 U/L (normal < 200 U/L). A muscle biopsy shows the characteristic findings of muscle fiber necrosis and size variability, as well as absent dystrophin on staining. Detection of deletions in the dystrophin gene using PCR is positive for 1 of the 21 regions studied.

Thought Questions

- What is the most likely diagnosis?
- What is the inheritance pattern of this disease?
- How would you counsel the parents on the risk to future children?
- What is the prognosis for this patient?

Basic Science Review and Discussion

Syndrome Description   Muscular dystrophy is the name for a group of inherited genetic disorders characterized by progressive muscle weakness and atrophy. The most common and most severe subtype is **Duchenne's muscular dystrophy (DMD).** This disease is an X-linked recessive disorder in which males are affected and females are asymptomatic carriers. The clinical symptoms usually begin before 5 years of age and include muscle weakness (proximal more than distal), clumsiness, pseudohypertrophy of the calves (due to fatty infiltration of the muscle), muscle contractures, and frequently mild mental retardation. The disease is rapidly progressive, and patients are usually wheelchair-bound by age 11 or 12. Eventually, the respiratory tract and cardiac muscles also weaken, and death occurs in the late teens or early 20s because of either pneumonia or cardiac dysfunction.

The diagnosis can be confirmed by an elevated serum creatine kinase level, an enzyme found in muscle and released into the serum upon muscle damage. Other diagnostic tests include electromyography to rule out a neuropathic disorder and a characteristic muscle biopsy showing fiber necrosis and size variation, as well as replacement of muscle by fat and connective tissue. Staining of the fibers shows a deficiency of dystrophin. There is currently no effective treatment to cure the disease, but a patient's life span can sometimes be extended to the late 20s with an elective tracheostomy and mechanical ventilatory support.

Genetics   In autosomal disorders, the disease's gene is located on one of the 22 pairs of non-sex chromosomes. In sex-linked disorders, the gene is inherited either on the X or on the Y chromosome. Most sex-linked diseases are found on the X chromosome and include recessive disorders like muscular dystrophy, hemophilia, and red-green color blindness. In females, an X-linked recessive disease acts like an AR disorder because both of the X chromosomes need to contain mutations for the phenotype to be manifested. In males, the disease has AD characteristics because the disorder will be manifested if the sole X chromosome contains the mutation. The Y chromosome does not contain most of the genes on the X chromosome and so is not protective. Remember that even in females, only one X chromosome will be expressed in each somatic cell (the other X chromo-

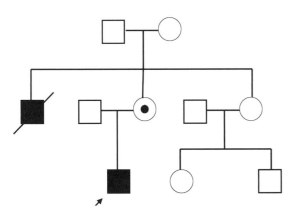

Figure 23-1

some is dormant because of X chromosome inactivation). In most diseases, a normal gene expression in 50% of the somatic cells is enough to either avoid the disease trait or have a milder version. However, when random chance causes the mutated chromosome to be active in an unexpectedly large number of cells **(skewed X inactivation)**, the disease trait can be seen in a female who is known as a **manifesting heterozygote.**

The **DMD gene** is one of the largest found in the human genome. It encodes for the dystrophin protein, which helps form a link between intracellular actin and the extracellular matrix. The characteristic pedigree of a family with an X-linked recessive disorder will normally show asymptomatic female carriers and affected males. In the most common situation when a female carrier has children, she is likely to pass the diseased allele to half her children. This means that half of her daughters will have a normal genotype and the other half will be asymptomatic carriers. Of her sons, half will be normal and the other half will show the traits of the disorder. The offspring of an affected male will be normal if they are male because they inherit the Y chromosome from their affected father, whereas the female offspring will all be carriers.

Case Conclusion WL's parents want to give him a normal childhood and enroll him in the local elementary school and high school. However, as time goes on, his ambulating difficulties become more incapacitating because of the worsening heel tendon contractures and his frequent collapses from leg weakness. Despite surgery to release the contractures, WL becomes confined to a wheelchair by age 12 years but is able to complete high school with the help of an electric wheelchair. In his late teens, he begins having breathing difficulties and elects to have a tracheostomy and assisted ventilation. He eventually dies of pneumonia at age 24.

Thumbnail: X-linked Recessive Genetics

X-linked Recessive Inheritance

X, normal X chromosome

x, mutant X chromosome

Carrier mother (Xx) and normal father (XY):

	X	x	
X	XX	xX	50% of daughters will be carriers
Y	XY	xY	50% of sons will be affected

Normal mother (XX) and affected father (xY):

	X	X	
x	xX	xX	100% of daughters will be carriers
Y	XY	XY	0% of sons will be affected

Key Points

- ▶ DMD is an X-linked recessive disorder.
- ▶ DMD is characterized by progressive proximal muscle weakness, muscle contractures, pseudohypertrophy of the calves, cardiac dysfunction, and recurrent pneumonias.
- ▶ Laboratory diagnosis involves elevated creatine kinase level, fatty infiltration of muscle, decreased dystrophin staining.
- ▶ X-linked disorders have asymptomatic female carriers and affected males.

Questions

1. WL's aunt (his mother's sister) is very worried about her son, who is 1 year old and so far asymptomatic. She would like to know what the chance is that she is also a carrier for the dystrophin gene deletion (Figure 23-2).

  A. 100%

  B. 66%

  C. 50%

  D. 25%

  E. 0%

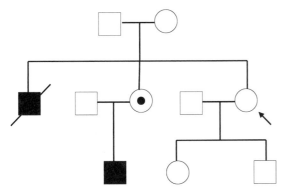

Figure 23-2

2. After extensive genetic testing, no mutations could be found in WL's male cousin, but his aunt and female cousin are found to be heterozygous for a deletion in the dystrophin gene. If WL marries his female cousin, what is the chance that their first daughter will be an asymptomatic carrier (Figure 23-3)?

  A. 100%

  B. 66%

  C. 50%

  D. 25%

  E. 0%

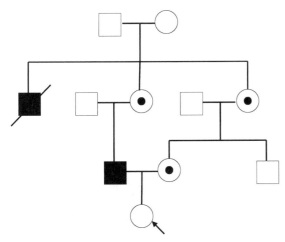

Figure 23-3

3. Assuming WL's grandfather died at a young age from an accident and nothing is known about his medical history, what are the chances that WL's grandmother is a carrier of DMD (Figure 23-4)?

  A. 100%

  B. 66%

  C. 50%

  D. 25%

  E. 0%

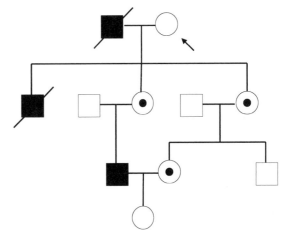

Figure 23-4

4. A 7-year-old boy is being seen in the ED for extensive bruising of the arms and legs after a fall. The parents state that their son had extensive bleeding during circumcision and is prone to bruises and swollen joints. The boy's grandfather had similar problems throughout his life and several male cousins are also affected. Which of the following statements is true about this disease?

  A. It has an X-linked dominant inheritance pattern.

  B. Platelet activity is abnormal.

  C. Men cannot pass the mutation to their daughters.

  D. There is deficient or defective factor VIII.

  E. There is deficient or defective factor VIII carrier protein.

HPI: TR is a 10-year-old boy with moderate mental retardation and autistic-like behavior. His parents first noted that he was "kind of slow" at 1 year of age, when he was not achieving his developmental milestones. He has an IQ of 68. On physical examination, he has nondysmorphic features, with average height and weight for his age. His initial newborn screening was normal. His parents are both healthy, of average intelligence, and nonconsanguineous. The family tree is shown in Figure 24-1, with an extensive family history of mental retardation, as you can see. TR has come to see you at the request of his new pediatrician for diagnostic evaluation. As part of the work-up for his mental retardation, you ordered chromosome analysis, which showed a normal 46,XY karyotype.

Thought Questions

- What type of inheritance pattern is suggested by the pedigree? Why?
- What is the molecular basis of fragile X syndrome?
- What is the phenotype of affected males and females with fragile X?

Basic Science Review and Discussion

The family tree depicted is somewhat atypical. It does not follow classic mendelian inheritance. Fragile X was initially thought to be X-linked recessive, but two observations did not conform with this pattern; 30% to 50% of carrier females had some degree of mental retardation, a proportion much higher than anticipated by X-linked recessive, and the fact that normal males could pass a mutant allele to their daughters who were also normal but were at risk of having mentally retarded sons. This unusual pattern was not well understood until the molecular basis was revealed.

Unstable DNA Triplet Repeat Sequences There are a number of disorders in which the mutation is an expansion of a triplet nucleotide repeat sequence that is unstable and can change in size on transmission from parent to offspring, sometimes called a **dynamic mutation.** Triple repeat DNA sequences are present throughout the human genome, and unstable triplet repeats constitute dynamic mutations that account for at least seven disorders known to humans (see Thumbnail: X-linked Dominant Inheritance). In general, the longer the repeat, the more likely it is to expand further on transmission. Also, the longer the repeat, the more severe

the phenotype (in AD disorders). Premutations are expansions of triple repeats beyond the normal range and are associated with a normal phenotype but can be unstable and expand to a full mutation associated with the disease phenotype, on transmission from parent to offspring.

Fragile X is caused by an **unstable CGG repeat** in the 5′ untranslated region of the **FMR1** gene on the X chromosome. In the normal population, the size of the repeat varies from 6 to 50 and remains stable (i.e., does not expand) from one generation to the next. Expansion from premutation to full mutation only occurs when the premutation is transmitted by females. Expansions of 60 to 200 repeats are considered a premutation. The larger the size of the premutation, the greater the chance of expanding into the full mutation range (>200). A mother carrying a premutation in the 60- to 69-repeat range has a chance of transmitting the premutation to a normal transmitting son, or it may expand to the full mutation range and she will have an affected son (8.5% risk). When the premutation is 90 or more repeats, the chance of expansion to full mutation is close to 100%.

Fragile X Phenotype Affected boys are mentally retarded in the moderate to severe range and often have autistic features. Speech tends to be halting and repetitive. Older boys and young adult men with the full mutation usually have discrete but recognizable physical features including a high forehead, long face, prominent jaw, and large ears. After puberty, most boys develop macro-orchidism. Females with the full mutation are mentally retarded about 30% to 50% of the time, usually in the mild to moderate range. Their physical features are not as clearly defined as those of their male counterparts.

Case Conclusion TR's parents decide to undergo DNA testing for fragile X syndrome. Southern blot of DNA from TR shows an expansion of the CGG triplet repeat of 600 (full mutation). His mother is a premutation carrier of 98 repeats. His parents are counseled about the risks of disease in future pregnancies, and TR is enrolled at a special-needs school that is better designed for his specific skill levels.

Thumbnail: X-linked Dominant Inheritance

Triplet Repeat Sequences

Syndrome/Disease	Inheritance pattern	Anticipation	Parental sex bias for instability	Repeat
Fragile X	X-linked dominant Partial penetrance in females	Yes	large expansion only maternal origin	CGG
Spinobulbar muscular atrophy	X-linked recessive	No	predominantly paternal	CAG
Myotonic dystrophy	AD	Yes	No	CTG
Huntington's disease	AD	Yes, but rare	Paternal	CAG
Spinocerebellar ataxia 1	AD	Yes	Unknown	CAG

Premutation can expand to full mutation only when passed mother → offspring

Key Points

Regarding Fragile X syndrome:

▶ Most common form of inherited mental retardation: 1 in 2000.

▶ X-linked dominant inheritance: About one third to one half of females with the full mutation are mentally retarded.

▶ Phenotype: Mild facial dysmorphisms and large testes after puberty. No obvious phenotype in affected females.

Questions

1. What are the chances of TR's sister having an affected daughter with fragile X syndrome?
   - **A.** 1 in 2
   - **B.** 1 in 4
   - **C.** 1 in 8
   - **D.** 1 in 16
   - **E.** She cannot have an affected daughter

2. TR's maternal uncle is a carrier of a premutation containing 70 triple repeats. What are the risks for his son and daughter of having mentally retarded offspring?
   - **A.** They are not at risk because their father does not have fragile X.
   - **B.** Both his son and his daughter are at risk of having mentally retarded children.
   - **C.** His daughter is at risk of having mentally retarded sons.
   - **D.** His daughter is at risk of having mentally retarded sons and daughters.
   - **E.** Too high, they should adopt children instead.

3. Triplet repeat DNA expansions represent a newly recognized type of mutation. This type of mutation can explain which of the following concepts?
   - **A.** Unusual pedigree patterns and anticipation
   - **B.** Genetic heterogeneity and gene dose effect
   - **C.** X-linked dominant inheritance and imprinting
   - **D.** Founder effect and heterozygote advantage
   - **E.** A and C are correct

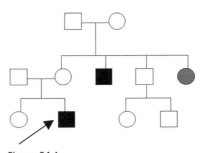

Figure 24-1

HPI: A 33-year-old woman is brought by ambulance to the ED with a complaint of hemiparesis and vision "blackout." She is well known to the ED staff and has been seen multiple times for similar strokelike episodes that resolve over a period of days. Her husband states that these episodes have been occurring with increasing frequency for the past 3 years. He has also noticed personality changes since the strokes began with increasing forgetfulness and irritability. The patient's medical history is significant for short stature, slight hearing deficit, frequent migraine headaches, and for becoming easily exhausted with mild exercise. She is an elementary school teacher but has been unable to work for the past year because of her constant fatigue. There is no family history of strokes, but the husband notes that her mother, an aunt, and an uncle frequently complain of low stamina and mild weakness. Interestingly, her aunt's children (cousins) also complain of these symptoms, but her uncle's children do not.

PE: The patient is somnolent, but arousable. HEENT exam reveals right-sided hemianopia and mild bilateral hearing deficit. On neurologic exam, she has mild muscle atrophy and decreased tone in all extremities. She is unable to move her right side against gravity and has proximal muscle weakness of the left side. The remainder of her exam is normal.

Labs: Serum lactic acid level is elevated at 6 mmol/L (normal < 2 mmol/L). A brain magnetic resonance imaging (MRI) scan shows lucency consistent with an infarct, as well as ventricular enlargement and occipital cortical atrophy. A Gomori trichome stain of a muscle biopsy reveals an intense red color, suggestive of mitochondrial accumulation.

Thought Questions

- What condition is suggested by this clinical presentation?
- What is the likely inheritance pattern?
- Why is this disease presenting at a later age?
- What is the prognosis for this patient?

Basic Science Review and Discussion

Syndrome Description The symptoms are consistent with a disease caused by mitochondrial DNA mutations. In this case, the patient was found to have **m**itochondrial myopathy, **e**ncephalopathy, **l**actic **a**cidosis, and **s**trokelike syndrome (collectively called **MELAS**). Like most other mitochondrial disorders, this disease has a complex set of symptoms characteristically involving the CNS and muscle. These two organs have high-energy consumption and are very sensitive to any disruption to mitochondrial ATP production. Patients with MELAS may have a normal childhood, but in early adulthood, they will experience easy fatigability, exercise intolerance, strokelike episodes with hemiplegia and vision changes, migrainelike headaches, seizures, and a progressive encephalopathy leading to dementia. Other associated symptoms include hearing loss, short stature, and diabetes.

The clinical diagnosis can be confirmed by **serum lactic acidosis** and a characteristic muscle biopsy showing a **"ragged red"** appearance from extensive mitochondrial proliferation. The biopsy sample can also be tested for decreased activity of mitochondrial respiratory chain enzymes, and

mitochondrial DNA mutation analysis can be done on either a blood sample or a muscle biopsy sample. The prognosis is poor, and the disease frequently results in mental deterioration with eventual dementia. There are currently no proven therapies, and treatment is generally supportive.

Mitochondrial Genetics Each human cell contains hundreds (or more) of mitochondria in the cytoplasm. Each mitochondrion in turn has multiple copies of **a circular double-stranded genome (mtDNA)**. In addition to the enzymes needed for oxidative phosphorylation, mitochondrial DNA also encodes for ribosomal and transfer RNAs that allow the mitochondria to produce proteins and to replicate independent of the nucleus. Although most genetic diseases are caused by mutations in the nuclear genome, an increasing number have been found to be due to mitochondrial defects. There are three different types of mitochondrial DNA mutations, which are used to classify the disorders. These include missense mutations, causing an amino acid substitution in the resulting protein (e.g., LHON). A second type of mtDNA mutation involves point mutations in a tRNA gene (e.g., MELAS), causing deficiencies in protein synthesis. The final class involves duplications and deletions (e.g., Kearns-Sayre syndrome) of the mitochondrial genome. There are three major differences between mitochondrial genetics and mendelian genetics: a maternal inheritance pattern, heteroplasmy/threshold effect, and replicative segregation.

Maternal Inheritance Pattern Because mitochondria are found in the cytoplasm, the fertilized embryo receives most of its mitochondria from the egg and little from the relatively small sperm cytoplasm. In addition, the mtDNA of the sperm is actively degraded after fertilization. Therefore, mitochondrial mutations are inherited only from mother to offspring. Although a male can be affected by a mitochondrial disorder, he is unable to pass the mutation to his children. This inheritance pattern is seen only in mitochondrial diseases.

Heteroplasmy and Threshold Effect   Because a mitochondrion contains multiple copies of its genome, each mitochondrion (and therefore each cell) can contain a mixture of normal mtDNA and mutated mtDNA. The ability of a cell to be composed of several types of mtDNA is known as **heteroplasmy.** In most situations, the severity of the disease increases with an increasing proportion of mutant mtDNA to normal mtDNA. There is a threshold for the proportion of mutant mtDNA, below which mitochondrial function remains normal, but above which function

becomes impaired. Therefore, a patient will not become symptomatic until a minimal number of mutant mtDNA is reached. This threshold of mutant mtDNA numbers needed for cellular dysfunction is lower in tissue with a high ATP requirement. For example, the CNS and muscle are highly dependent on oxidative phosphorylation and so are two of the most severely affected organs.

Replicative Segregation   As mitochondria divide, the proportion of mutant to wild-type mtDNA changes. This phenomenon is known as **replicative segregation.** This process can occur either through chance or by a selective advantage of one mtDNA species over another. Over time, this process may cause the proportion of mutant mtDNA to increase past the threshold, leading to the unmasking of the disease phenotype. This may contribute to the delayed onset of the symptoms seen in the mitochondrial disorders.

Case Conclusion   Mitochondrial DNA mutation analysis shows that the patient has an A-to-G substitution at nucleotide 3243 of the tRNA gene. This is the most common mutation seen in the MELAS syndrome and is found in 80% of affected individuals. After consultation with a geneticist, the patient and her husband decide to forgo having any children because of the high likelihood of passing the mutation on to any offspring. Her dementia worsens over the next few years, and she is finally placed in a nursing facility when her husband becomes unable to care for her.

Thumbnail: Mitochondrial Inheritance

Mitochondrial Genetics

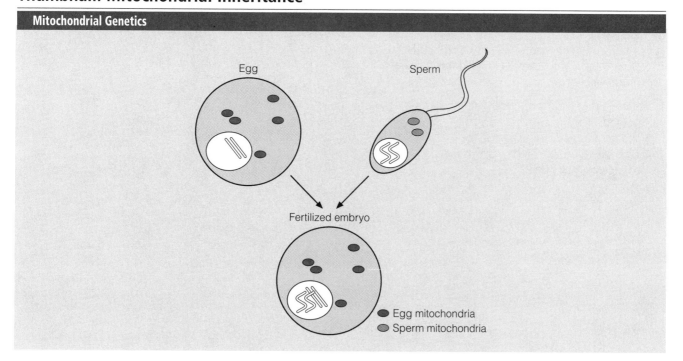

Key Points

▶ MELAS is caused by a mitochondrial DNA mutation.

▶ Key organs affected by MELAS include muscle (exercise intolerance, lactic acidosis) and the CNS (strokelike episodes, seizures, encephalopathy).

▶ Laboratory diagnosis involves serum lactic acidosis, muscle biopsy showing red ragged fibers, and DNA mutation analysis (3243A→G mutation most common).

▶ Mitochondrial genetics differ from mendelian genetics in three aspects:

1. Maternal inheritance: Affected males cannot transmit a mitochondrial disorder.

2. Heteroplasmy: multiple mtDNA species are found in a cell or tissue.

3. Replicative segregation: As cells and mitochondria divide and proliferate, the proportion of mutant mtDNA to wild-type mtDNA can change.

Questions

1. MELAS is transmitted via a mitochondrial inheritance pattern. It has similarities to both autosomal and sex-linked inheritance. Which of the following is true of both mitochondrial and X-linked recessive inheritance?

   A. Only females can transmit the gene to the next generation.
   B. Males are more likely than females to be affected (have symptoms).
   C. Females are more likely than males to be affected (have symptoms).
   D. No offspring of an affected male can be affected (have symptoms) if the female has normal genotype.
   E. All offspring of an affected female will show symptoms of the disease, assuming the male has a normal genotype.

2. Assuming that the mitochondrial mutation was not de novo and all of the branches on a particular pedigree are blood related, what is the probability that a maternal aunt of an individual affected with MELAS will also have the mitochondrial mutation?

   A. 100%
   B. 75%
   C. 50%
   D. 25%
   E. 0%

3. There are several differences between mtDNA and cell nuclear DNA. With the exception of the sex chromosomes, human nuclear DNA normally have two copies of each chromosome while hundreds (or thousands) of mitochondrial DNA may be present. Which of the following terms describes the ability of a cell to have multiple different populations of mtDNA?

   A. Threshold effect
   B. Heteroplasmy
   C. Homoplasmy
   D. Pleiotropy
   E. Imprinting

HPI: A 10-month-old girl is referred to you by her pediatrician for a growth in her back. The mother states that the mass was first noticed 3 months ago and has been growing slowly since then. She reports that the patient has fallen behind on her developmental milestones (she is still unable to crawl or sit without support) but denies any other significant medical problems. The only significant family history is the patient's 5-year-old brother, who has decreased vision in his right eye.

PE: The patient is an alert infant with normal weight and growth. HEENT exam reveals multiple scattered nodules on the left iris (Lisch nodules). She has numerous 5- to 10-mm hyperpigmented patches (café au lait macules) over her trunk and extremities, as well as freckling of the axillary and inguinal regions. A 4 × 5-cm firm, immobile mass is found left of the midline on her back. The remainder of her exam shows no abnormalities.

Labs: CT of the spine shows a large homogeneous enhancing mass at the level of T4-T5. An MRI of the brain shows no tumors.

Thought Questions

- What is the most likely diagnosis?
- What is the inheritance pattern of this disease?
- Why might this patient have presented with a "negative" family history?
- What is the genetic basis of this disease?

Basic Science Review and Discussion

Syndrome Description **Neurofibromatosis type 1 (NF1)** is an **AD** disorder affecting 1 in 3000 individuals. NF1 has a highly variable expression of symptoms, but features generally include **café au lait spots** (describing the hyperpigmented macules), **axillary/inguinal freckling, Lisch nodules** (benign growths on the iris), **neurofibromas** (benign proliferation of Schwann cells around peripheral nerves), **optic gliomas,** and **bone lesions** (scoliosis, vertebral dysplasia). Other symptoms may include learning disability, epilepsy, and hypertension. Because NF1 is an AD disease, it affects equal proportions of males and females, shows no skipped generations, and has male-to-male transmission.

Diagnosis is made clinically with imaging frequently finding optic gliomas, neurofibromas, and CNS hamartomas. Most patients do not require treatment, but disfiguring or painful peripheral neurofibromas can be removed surgically.

Variable Expression and Penetrance The clinical presentation of NF1 can be highly variable, even between affected members of a family. Most patients have only mild cutaneous involvement—café au lait spots and few neurofibromas. However, those who are severely affected may have many if not all of the aforementioned symptoms, including hun-

dreds or thousands of neurofibromas. The multiple potential manifestations of a disease phenotype is termed **variable expression.** Although the exact cause remains unclear in the case of NF1, variable expression in general can be attributed to environmental effects, interactions with other genes (modifier genes), or different types of mutations at a single disease gene locus (allelic heterogeneity).

Reduced penetrance is the concept that an individual with a disease genotype may not always have the resulting disease phenotype, even though the individual is able to transmit the mutation to the next generation. The disease manifestation is not categorized based on severity but is seen as all or nothing. One example of this concept can be seen in **retinoblastoma** in which one copy of the Rb1 tumor suppressor gene becomes nonfunctional due to a mutation. If the other copy of this gene also acquires a mutation during the lifetime of the individual, then the disease phenotype (malignant intraocular tumors) will be seen. This second mutation does not occur in 10% of patients, who remain disease-free throughout their lifetime. Thus, the penetrance of the Rb1 gene is said to be 90%.

Pleiotropy and Locus Heterogeneity NF is caused by genetic mutations in the neurofibromin gene on chromosome 17. The gene product acts as a tumor suppressor, but in addition to benign and malignant growths, mutations in this gene can also cause a variety of other symptoms including learning disabilities, hypertension, and bone defects. This is an example of **pleiotropy,** the ability of a gene to influence multiple phenotypes. Pleiotropy is involved in myriad other diseases including **Marfan's syndrome,** a connective tissue abnormality that leads to defects in the ocular, skeletal, and cardiovascular systems.

Although a gene can have several disease phenotypes, one disease phenotype can also be caused by mutations in multiple different genes. This is known as **locus heterogeneity** and can be seen in diseases such as adult polycystic kidney disease (APKD). APKD can be caused by mutations in genes on either chromosome 16 **(PKD1)** or chromosome 4

(PKD2). These two genes produce membrane glycoproteins that interact with each other, and a defect in either will lead to a progressive accumulation of renal cysts, which are characteristic of this disease.

Case Conclusion The patient eventually undergoes an elective resection of the mass, which is determined by the pathologist to be a benign schwannoma, confirming the diagnosis of NF. The patient's father and brother are reexamined and several scattered café au lait spots are found on their trunk and back. The brother is referred to an ophthalmologist who finds multiple Lisch nodules and an optic nerve glioma, causing the decreased vision in his right eye.

Thumbnail: Variable Penetrance

Key Principles of Medical Genetics

Genetic principle	Definition	Examples
Variable expression	Variation in the severity of a disease due to environmental effects, allelic heterogeneity, or interaction with other (modifier) genes	NF1, osteogenesis imperfecta
Allelic heterogeneity	Variable expression of a disease phenotype based on type of mutation at a disease locus	Osteogenesis imperfecta
Reduced penetrance	When having a disease genotype does not necessarily produce the disease phenotype	Retinoblastoma
Pleiotropy	Ability of a gene to cause many phenotypes	NF1, Marfan's syndrome, CF
Locus heterogeneity	When mutations at different gene loci can cause the same disease phenotype	APKD

Key Points

▶ NF1 is an AD disorder caused by a mutation in the neurofibromin tumor suppressor gene.

▶ NF1 is characterized by café au lait spots, axillary/inguinal freckling, Lisch nodules, neurofibromas, optic gliomas, and bone lesions. Associated symptoms include hypertension, developmental delay, and malignancies.

▶ Reasons for a "negative" family history in a patient with an inheritable disease are as follows:

1. New mutation
2. Variable expression
3. Reduced penetrance
4. Wrong diagnosis
5. False paternity

Questions

1. Osteogenesis imperfecta is a class of inherited diseases with varying severity, but all are characterized by abnormalities in the formation of the bone matrix, leading to an increased risk of fractures. It has been discovered that one possible cause for the highly variable symptoms is the location of the mutation in the gene. Mutations at the C-terminus of the procollagen gene result in more severe symptoms than those at the amino-terminal. This scenario is embodied by which genetic concept?

   A. Reduced penetrance
   B. Imprinting
   C. Pleiotropy
   D. Variable expression
   E. Anticipation

2. Multiple members of a single family are seen in your office with several presentations of a single disease. The mildest cases have only the dermatologic findings of hypopigmented "ash-leaf spots," fibromas of the nail, and *shagreen patches* (leather-textured area of subepidermal fibrosis normally found on the back). The most severe cases have the additional symptoms of seizures, mental retardation, and facial angiofibromas (vascular tumors). What is the most likely diagnosis of this inheritable disease?

   A. Sturge-Weber syndrome
   B. NF2
   C. von Recklinghausen's disease
   D. Marfan's syndrome
   E. Tuberous sclerosis

3. Myotonic dystrophy is an AD disorder characterized by facial and extremity muscle weakness, cataracts, intellectual impairment, and abnormalities in the respiratory, GI, and cardiac systems. This disease is caused by a CTG trinucleotide expansion in a gene on chromosome 19. Recently, a family with myotonic dystrophy was found to have a mutation on chromosome 3 instead. The symptoms exhibited by members of this family are indistinguishable from those caused by the chromosome 19 mutation. Which of the following terms defines the ability of a disease to be caused by mutations at different gene loci in different families?

   A. Pleiotropy
   B. Allelic heterogeneity
   C. Locus heterogeneity
   D. Heteroplasmy
   E. Reduced or incomplete penetrance

HPI: You are a medical student rotating through the pediatrics service and your first day is in the acute care clinic. Your first patient is TS, an 8-month-old white male infant who is brought in by his teenage mother. His mother is a first-time mom living in a teen home and tells you that her baby just does not seem right. He is not very alert and seems to be "jumpy" with noises. She is also worried because he seems slower than the other 8-month-old babies at the program. She reports that TS's prenatal care was normal, except that she started care late, at 30 weeks. The delivery was normal as well.

PE: It is obvious that TS is neurologically impaired. He lacks muscle tone and is delayed in motor and intellectual milestones. The head and neck exam are normal, except that on funduscopic exam, you astutely notice a cherry-red spot. The cardiac, pulmonary, and abdominal exams show no abnormalities. You present this patient to the attending physician and your plan is to order a hexosaminidase A (Hex A) serum level.

Thought Questions

■ What enzyme deficiency causes Tay-Sachs disease and how does its absence lead to the disease?

■ What types of mutation lead to the disease?

■ What kind of prenatal counseling and genetic screening can be done? Who should be screened?

Basic Science Review and Discussion

Tay-Sachs disease is an **AR** disease that is most commonly seen in eastern European Jews and French Canadians. Approximately 1 in 27 Ashkenazi Jews is a carrier for the Tay-Sachs allele, making the incidence of the disease in this population 100 times greater than that in other populations. It is thought that this is due to either a **founder effect,** in which the high frequency of a mutant gene in a population is founded by a small ancestral group when one or more founders is a carrier for the mutation, or a **heterozygote advantage,** in which being heterozygote for the mutation offers a selection advantage over both homozygous genotypes.

The classic example of heterozygote advantage is the resistance to malaria in individuals heterozygous for sickle-cell anemia. The RBCs in these individuals function in normal conditions but are inhospitable to *Plasmodium vivax,* the parasitic protozoan responsible for malaria. Normal homozygotes are susceptible to malaria, and sickle cell homozygotes are more seriously disadvantaged by their disease. The heterozygotes, whose RBCs are adequate in normal conditions and are resistant to malarial infections, have a survival advantage, and therefore, with time, the sickle gene has been propagated and reached high frequencies in malaria endemic areas.

Infants with Tay-Sachs **develop symptoms at 3 to 10 months of age.** These symptoms include a loss of alertness and an excessive reaction to noise **(hyperacusis).** There is a **progressive neurologic degeneration** with developmental delay in intellectual and neurologic function. One to three months later, myoclonic and akinetic seizures can present. One physical exam finding is the cherry-red spots seen on the funduscopic eye exam, where the prominent red macular fovea centralis is contrasted by the pale macula. These children eventually suffer from paralysis, blindness, and dementia, and die by 4 years of age.

Tay-Sachs Pathophysiology   The disease is due to the deficiency of **Hex A,** the enzyme responsible for the degradation of G_{M2} gangliosides. Hex A is a multimeric protein composed of three parts: an α and β subunit that comprises the enzyme and an activator protein. The activator protein must associate with both the enzyme and the substrate before it can cleave the ganglioside between the *N*-acetyl-β-galactosamine and galactose residues. Gangliosides are continually degraded in lysosomes where multiple degradative enzymes function to sequentially remove the terminal sugars off the gangliosides. The impact of Tay-Sachs disease is mainly in the brain, where gangliosides are found in the highest concentration, particularly in the gray matter. The deficiency of Hex A results in the accumulations of gangliosides in the lysosomes, resulting in enlarged neurons containing lipid-filled lysosomes, cellular dysfunction, and ultimately neuronal death.

Although mutations that affect any part of the multimeric protein can lead to disease, Tay-Sachs disease occurs with a **mutation in the α subunit of Hex A,** whose locus is located on band 15q23-q24. Mutations in the β subunit lead to Sandhoff's disease and defects in the activator protein lead to activator deficiency. There are multiple single-gene mutations that lead to the disease, but there are only two common ones. The first involves a 4-base pair (bp) insertion into exon 11, resulting in a **premature stop codon.** This form is seen in approximately 79% of the Ashkenazi Jews. The second mutation is an **error in RNA splicing** in exon 12, resulting in the substitution of a cytosine from a guanine, and this is seen in approximately 18% of Ashkenazi Jews. Of note, there is an adult-onset form of Tay-Sachs disease, and this is differentiated from the infantile forms in that there is a small amount of functioning enzyme and the age at onset is roughly proportional to the amount of residual activity.

There is **no cure** for Tay-Sachs disease. Genetic counseling and prenatal diagnosis, however, can be offered for any couples at risk, particular those of Jewish heritage. **Amniocentesis** or **CVS** can be done to obtain fetal cells that can be used for DNA and enzyme activity analysis.

Case Conclusion   TS has Hex A level drawn and the enzyme is found to be absent. TS is diagnosed with Tay-Sachs disease and is followed closely by a pediatric neurologist. There is no treatment for this disease. As expected, he has a neurologically degenerating course and dies at age 3 years.

Thumbnail: Tay-Sachs Molecular Biology

The active Hex A molecule is composed of three gene products and a defect in any of these products can lead to disease. Deficiency in the α subunit, which is found on chromosome 15, leads to Tay-Sachs disease and late-onset variants. Sandhoff's disease and similar late-onset variants are due to a defect in the β subunit, and this is encoded on chromosome 5. The errors in these two forms result in a defective enzyme complex. A deficiency in the activator, encoded on chromosome 5, leads to activator deficiency and an overall lack in Hex A activity.

Key Points

▶ Tay-Sachs disease is more common in Ashkenazi Jews, possibly because of a founder effect or heterozygote advantage.

▶ Tay-Sachs disease is due to a deficiency in Hex A, resulting in the inability to degrade G_{M2} ganglioside, accumulation of gangliosides in neurons, and subsequently neuronal cell death.

▶ Hex A exists as a multimer consisting of an enzyme with an α and β subunit, as well as an activator protein.

▶ Tay-Sachs disease is due to single-gene defects in the α-subunit locus, two of the most common being a premature stop codon and the other an RNA splicing error.

▶ Genetic counseling and prenatal diagnosis, which include amniocentesis or CVS, should be offered to couples at risk of Tay-Sachs disease.

Questions

1. Theoretically, why might Tay-Sachs disease be more prevalent in the Ashkenazi Jewish population?

   A. Because of the high frequency of consanguinity in this population

   B. Because it is transmitted in an AD fashion

   C. Because of the possibility of a heterozygote advantage

   D. Because a mutation in any protein of the Hex A multimer, either the α or β subunit or the activator protein, can cause the disease

   E. Because of mitochondrial inheritance

2. Tay-Sachs disease is an AR genetic disorder. What is the genetic defect responsible for Tay-Sachs disease?

   A. Inversion

   B. Recombination error

   C. Translocation

   D. Single-gene mutation

   E. Gene deletion

3. An Ashkenazi Jewish woman that is 16 weeks pregnant presents for genetic counseling and requests an amniocentesis to test for Tay-Sachs disease. What in the amniotic fluid do you test for?

   A. G_{M2} ganglioside activity

   B. Sphingomyelinase activity

   C. Glucocerebroside activity

   D. Hex A activity

   E. Arylsulfatase A activity

HPI: You are called from the well-baby nursery to evaluate JL, a full-term newborn who is having difficulty feeding and latching 1 day after delivery. He was born to a 32-year-old mother, first pregnancy, which was uneventful. The maternal serum prenatal screening revealed a risk for Down syndrome of 1 in 180, but his parents declined amniocentesis after genetic counseling and a normal obstetric ultrasound (US) at 18 weeks. JL was delivered by uncomplicated vaginal delivery, at 40 and 3/7 weeks. He weighed 3.3 kg, was 51 cm long, and had a head circumference of 50 cm at birth. His Apgar scores were 7 and 9 at 1 and 5 minutes, respectively.

PE: JL has marked hypotonia, and a poor Moro's reflex. You also notice a flat facial profile, mid-facial hypoplasia, a rounded head, and a special appearance of his eyes, particularly when he is crying. His tongue appears too big for the size of the mouth. His neck is short with redundant loose skin. He has clinodactyly of the fifth fingers and a wide sandal groove of the toes. You are also concerned about a grade 3/6 pansystolic heart murmur.

Thought Questions

- What is the most likely diagnosis?

- What are the clinical features of this disorder?

- Why is confirmation of the diagnosis so important?

- What is the etiology of this condition?

Basic Science Review and Discussion

Syndrome Description DS is the most common cause of genetic mental retardation, with an incidence of 1 in 1000 live births. In the newborn period, severe hypotonia and lethargy are the norm. A combination of associated minor anomalies, none of which is specific or pathognomonic, gives affected individuals a specific recognizable appearance. Craniofacial features include brachycephaly, flat facial profile, upslanted palpebral fissures, epicanthic folds, protruding tongue in a small mouth, small simple ears, and loose redundant neck skin. Skeletal findings include single palmar crease, small middle phalanx of the fifth digit, hyperextensible large joints, wide gap between first and second toe, and short stature. Cardiac malformations are present in 40% of cases and have a significant impact on infant mortality. VSD, auricular septal defects, common atrioventricular canal, and patent ductus arteriosus are the most common heart defects. Other common major malformations include anal atresia and duodenal atresia. Hearing loss (both conductive and sensorineural) is common. Ocular anomalies (e.g., cataracts, strabismus, glaucoma, and major refractory errors) are also very common. Early recognition of hearing and visual impairment is essential because they may further accentuate the mental retardation if untreated. Mental retardation is universal in DS, with an IQ range of 25 to 75. Children with DS are generally happy, have good social skills, and are very affectionate. Most adults with DS develop early onset Alzheimer's disease. Life expectancy is 50 years in the United States.

Chromosome Findings Ninety-five percent of DS cases are a result of trisomy 21 (47,XX,+21 or 47,XY,+21 karyotype). The additional chromosome is of maternal origin 90% of the time, which arises as a result of **nondisjunction during maternal meiosis I.** There is a well-recognized maternal age effect and increased risk of **aneuploidy** (a chromosome number that is not an exact multiple of the haploid number). **Robertsonian translocations** account for 3% of DS cases, of which one third of the time one of the parents is found to be a balance carrier. These couples are at a significant risk of recurrence, which varies depending of the type of translocation and who is the carrier parent (i.e., male or female, with males transmitting an unbalanced complement less often). The rest of DS cases (2%) are due to mosaicism of trisomy 21. Individuals with mosaic trisomy 21 tend on average to have higher IQs than those with full trisomy. It is possible that the phenotype of DS (and other trisomies) is the result of an increased dose of specific genes on the extra chromosome. Chromosome analysis is essential in suspected cases of DS in order to confirm the diagnosis, provide accurate recurrence risk, and to a lesser degree provide some information about the prognosis (mosaic cases).

Case Conclusion After your assessment, you suspect that JL has DS. In a private setting, you meet with both of JL's parents and disclose your impressions and provide counseling. An echocardiogram showed a small VSD. Ophthalmology and hearing evaluations have been requested. Two days later, a FISH study using a fluorescent probe specific for chromosome 21 reveals an extra set in each of the 45 metaphases analyzed. Standard chromosome analysis reveals a 47,XY,+21 karyotype, confirming the diagnosis.

Thumbnail: Chromosome Structure

Nondisjunction Meiosis I

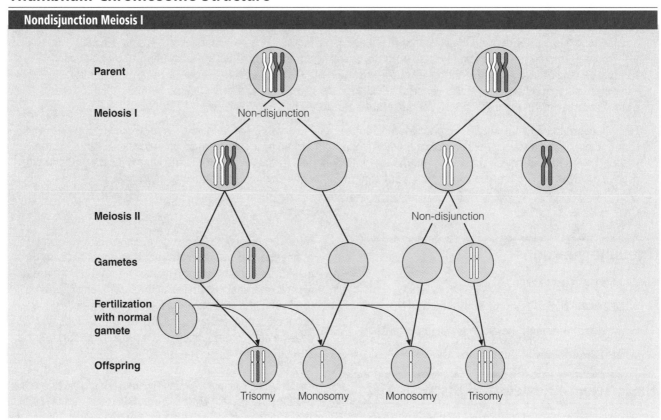

Key Points

- ▶ Most common genetic cause of mental retardation, 1 in 1000 live births
- ▶ DS: 95% trisomy 21, 3% translocation, 2% mosaic
- ▶ Most common trisomy: trisomy 16, but not compatible with life (all are spontaneous abortions)
- ▶ Maternal age effect: trisomy 21, trisomy 13, and trisomy 18
- ▶ Paternal age effect: increased incidence of spontaneous AD mutations (e.g., NF1, tuberous sclerosis [TS], and achondroplasia)

Questions

1. After confirmation of the diagnosis, you inform JL's parents that the recurrence risk in the next pregnancy is what?
   A. Same as maternal age risk
   B. 1% greater than expected for maternal age risk
   C. 10% to 12%
   D. 100%
   E. Cannot provide adequate recurrence risk

2. Three years later JL's parents are considering pregnancy and are interested in prenatal diagnosis. Upon discussion of the different modalities of invasive prenatal diagnosis, you explain which of the following?
   A. The incidence of diagnosing trisomy 21 is the same with CVS and amniocentesis.
   B. The incidence of diagnosing trisomy 21 is higher with CVS than amniocentesis.
   C. Amniocentesis has a higher pregnancy-related loss rate than CVS.
   D. Amniocentesis can be associated with confined placental mosaicism.
   E. A normal fetal US at 18 weeks rules out DS.

3. Children with DS are at an increased risk of which of the following medical complications?
   A. Acute lymphoblastic leukemia
   B. Epilepsy
   C. Hypothyroidism
   D. Atlantoaxial subluxation
   E. All of the above

HPI: RA is a 28-year-old woman who is G4 P0 S3 T1 (4 pregnancies, no births, 3 miscarriages, 1 abortion); she comes to your office for genetic counseling. She and her husband have been trying to get pregnant over the last year but have had three consecutive first-trimester miscarriages, which all occurred within the first 7 to 8 weeks of gestation. She had one therapeutic abortion at approximately 7 weeks when she was 17 years old for an undesired pregnancy. Her medical, surgical, and gynecologic history are unremarkable. She was adopted and has no information regarding her biologic parents or their families. Her husband has an unremarkable medical and family history.

Thought Questions

- What is the definition of recurrent or habitual abortions?

- What are some of the causes for these pregnancy losses?

- Describe the process of meiosis. What is nondisjunction?

Basic Science Review and Discussion

Genetics of Recurrent Abortions   Recurrent or habitual abortions is defined as **three consecutive pregnancy losses.** In roughly 50% of cases, no etiology for the loss is found. In the remainder of cases, the cause for the loss falls into six main categories: **genetic error, anatomic abnormalities of the reproductive tract, hormonal disfunction, infection, immunologic factors,** and **systemic diseases.** In the first and second trimesters, 15% of cases are due to infection and 12% cases are due to uterine defects. Cervical incompetence accounts for 3% of losses in the first trimester and 30% of second-trimester losses. Chromosomal abnormalities account for 4% to 10% of recurrent losses in the first trimester but very few in the second trimester. Systemic diseases in general cause only second-trimester losses and are seen approximately 3% of the time. In this review, we focus on the genetic causes of recurrent losses.

There is a 50% to 60% incidence of an **abnormal karyotype** in any spontaneous first-trimester abortion, but only a 7.3% incidence in planned abortions. These abnormalities are secondary to trisomies (52%), polyploidy (26%), X monosomy (15%), and occasional cases of double trisomies, mosaicisms, and translocations. Possible causes of genetic errors include translocations of parental chromosomes, chromosomal variations from recombination defects, biochemical disorders, environmental insults, viral infections, and delayed fertilization of an ovulated ovum.

Trisomy, the most common genetic aberrancy detected, typically is due to nondisjunction during the first meiotic division. Autosomal transmission of a trisomy also occurs and appears to be a nonrandom event. The trisomy can be transferred from either a maternal or a paternal source.

Carriers of balanced translocations have an increased risk of spontaneous abortions and karyotype abnormalities in their offspring.

Meiosis   To better understand how a nondisjunction event can occur, we review the steps of meiosis. Germ cells undergo cell division for the production of gametes by this process. During meiosis, a germ cell (for the production of either a sperm or an ovum), undergoes **two sets of divisions to reduce its chromosome number from 46 to 23,** converting from a normal diploid complement of chromosomes down to a haploid set. Each cell therefore contains only one member of each chromosome pair. Once fertilization occurs, the fusion of the two pronuclei from a sperm and an ovum reconstitutes to the diploid state.

Meiosis occurs in two major phases, meiosis I and meiosis II, and each phase is subdivided into many steps. In meiosis I, the first step is prophase I. During this time, the chromatin condenses and becomes a single elongated threadlike structure and migrates toward the equatorial plate of the nucleus. Homologous chromosomes become closely arranged to form "bivalents" that can exchange genetic information by **homologous recombination.** Afterward, the chromosomes further contract to become shorter and thicker. They split longitudinally into two chromatids connected at the centromere. The bivalents are held together at certain points on the chromosomes, called **bridges or chiasms.** These are the points at which **crossover events** take place. Next, the bivalents contract and the chiasms move toward the end of the chromosomes, the homologues separate, and the nuclear membranes disappear. In metaphase I, the bivalents realign at the equatorial plate. Next come anaphase I and telophase I, respectively, where the bivalent pair separates to each spindle but not the sister chromatids. The spindles then break down, and the cytoplasm divides to form two daughter cells.

Meiosis II follows next. During metaphase II, the chromosomes again align at the equatorial plate and then the chromatids divide at the centromeres. Anaphase II and telophase II occur, resulting in each daughter cell containing a haploid number of chromosomes. In spermatogenesis, the **spermatogonium produces four equal sperm.** In contrast, during oogenesis, only one egg is produced. With each division, two daughter cells are produced, each with an intact haploid complement. However, one daughter cell has very little cytoplasm secondary to an unequal cytoplasmic division. This small daughter cell is known as a *polar body.* One polar body is formed after both meiosis I and meiosis II. Therefore, each oogonium produces only one ovum.

Nondisjunction can occur in mitosis or meiosis. When nondisjunction occurs during mitosis, the chromosomes divide unequally and an extra chromatid can segregate to one of the daughter cells, with the other lacking that particular chromatid. After cell division, **one cell becomes trisomic and the other is monosomic.** When these cells continue to proliferate and establish a clonal line within the individual, it is known as **mosaicism.**

When nondisjunction occurs during meiosis, both chromosomes of a homologous pair segregate to one cell while the other has none. As a consequence, once an ovum containing a chromosome pair is fertilized, a trisomy will result. If an ovum that is missing a chromosome pair is fertilized, a monosomy will result. Depending on which chromosomes are involved, the trisomic or monosomic state may be lethal, resulting in an early spontaneous abortion. Aneuploidy of the sex chromosomes is not necessarily lethal, and examples of sex chromosome monosomy and trisomy have been documented.

Case Conclusion   A three-generation pedigree and karyotyping of both RA and her husband is performed. Karyotyping of the last abortus was also done. RA was found to be a carrier of a balanced translocation. Given this information, RA and her husband decided to proceed with in vitro fertilization with donation of ova from her sister.

Thumbnail: Translocation

Causes of Recurrent Pregnancy Losses	
Causes	**Examples**
1. Genetic error	Abnormal karyotypes, such as trisomy, monosomy, polyploidy
2. Abnormalities of the female reproductive tract	Congenital uterine anomalies, cervical incompetence, myomas, Asherman's syndrome
3. Hormonal deficiency	Hyperthyroidism, hypothyroidism, progesterone deficiency
4. Infection	Mycoplasma, toxoplasmosis, listeria, chlamydia, gonorrhea, herpes simplex, syphilis, CMV, brucella
5. Immunologic factors	Unclear, but increased sharing of the HLA-A and HLA-B between partners, fewer inhibitors of cell-mediated immunity, absence of transplant antigen
6. Systemic disease	Autoimmune diseases (e.g., SLE), diabetes, coagulopathies

---

Key Points

▶ Genetic abnormalities are typically due to chromosomal anomalies from nondisjunction events during meiosis.

▶ Meiosis occurs in two main phases: meiosis I and meiosis II. It is a multistep process that eventually results in the reduction of the chromosome content from diploid to haploid.

Questions

1. A 37-year-old woman who is G4 P1 T2 obtains a CVS (a technique to obtain chorionic villi for genetic analysis) at 11 weeks of gestation. Given her age, she had concerns of having a child with DS. Adequate tissue was obtained by an experienced provider and the results revealed both a normal karyotype of 46,XY, and an abnormal karyotype of 47,XY Trisomy 21. Four weeks later, she undergoes an amniocentesis, which reveals a normal 46,XY karyotype. The discrepancy between the CVS result and the amniocentesis is likely due to which of the following?

   A. Inadequate cellular differentiation for the determination of DS
   B. Confined placental mosaicism
   C. Nondisjunction during meiosis I
   D. Nondisjunction during meiosis II
   E. Paternal carrier not detected by CVS

2. At birth, the ova in a female infant are arrested in prophase I of the first meiotic division. The first meiotic division is completed just before ovulation. Immediately after this, meiosis II begins but is arrested in metaphase II. Completion of meiosis II can occur only upon fertilization. Which of the following describes metaphase II?

   A. Chromosomes condense to form a single elongated threadlike structure.
   B. Bivalents form and homologous recombination occurs.
   C. Chromosomes are held together at chiasms and crossover events occur.
   D. Chromosomes align at the equatorial plate.
   E. Chromatids pull apart and move toward each spindle.

3. Which is the correct order of events in meiosis I?

   A. Anaphase, prophase, metaphase, telophase
   B. Metaphase, prophase, telophase, anaphase
   C. Prophase, anaphase, metaphase, telophase
   D. Telophase, prophase, metaphase, anaphase
   E. Prophase, metaphase, anaphase, telophase

HPI: CA is a young female adolescent who has come to see you regarding her lack of sexual development. Unlike her two older sisters who initiated secondary sexual changes at age 10 and 11, CA at age 14 still has not shown any signs of secondary sexual development. You learn that CA is a B+ student in the eighth grade who works an inordinate amount of hours to achieve her grades. CA's mother notes that she has always been a bit clumsy and has not shown much interest in sports, particularly those involving hand-eye coordination. Recently, it appears that she has been experiencing some low self-esteem because of her short stature and "not changing like the other girls have."

PE: CA's height is at the fifth percentile and her weight is at the forty-fifth percentile for her age. Her facial appearance is unremarkable, but you do notice that her ears are a bit prominent and she has a low posterior hairline. There is mild posterior webbing of the neck. Cardiac exam including auscultation, BP readings of four extremities, and ECG is unremarkable. There is no evidence of secondary sexual development (Tanner's grade I). Her chest is broad with widely spaced nipples. She has normal yet immature external genitalia. The rest of the exam is noncontributory.

Thought Questions

- What is the most likely diagnosis?
- What are the clinical features of this disorder at different stages of life?
- What is the origin of the chromosomal defect?

Basic Science Review and Discussion

The most consistent feature in Turner's syndrome is short stature and gonadal dysgenesis. Because the manifestations of ovarian failure are not evident in childhood, chromosome studies should be pursued in any girl with short stature and whose phenotype is not incompatible with Turner's syndrome.

Syndrome Description The vast majority of concepti with Turner's syndrome will abort spontaneously. In the cases ascertained prenatally, fetal edema is commonly found, manifested as either increased nuchal translucency, nuchal edema, or generalized fetal edema (fetal hydrops). In the newborn period, congenital lymphedema with puffiness of the back of the neck, feet, and hands with hyperconvex nails as a result of the edema can be seen. Posterior webbing of the neck is common. The short stature is usually present from birth, although other manifestations can be present at any age. The thorax is broad with wide-spaced nipples. There can be subtle facial dysmorphisms—none of which is characteristic or pathognomonic—such as low posterior hairline and short neck appearance. Cubitus valgus is very common. Cardiac malformations, including bicuspid aortic valve (30%) and coarctation of the aorta (10%), should be ruled out. Delays in motor skills, poor coordination, and visuospatial organization problems are common, but most will have normal intelligence. Ovarian dysgenesis is present in more than 90%, manifesting as primary amenorrhea, but is *not* universal. A few girls with Turner's syndrome will undergo secondary sexual development, and even fewer have been known to conceive spontaneously. The few that have spontaneous onset of menses will often experience early premature ovarian failure.

Chromosome Findings The absence of a second sex chromosome is diagnostic of Turner's syndrome. This absence may be a deletion of part or all of either an X or a Y chromosome. Nearly half of patients with Turner's syndrome have monosomy X (45,X). Of these, 75% are due to the loss of either an X or a Y chromosome during paternal meiosis II. Other causes of Turner's syndrome include mosaicism (e.g., 45,X/46,XX), isochromosome 46,X,i(Xp) in which there is loss of one chromosome arm and duplication of the other, ring chromosome 46,X,r(X) where there is a break on each arm of the chromosome, leaving "sticky ends" that bind forming a ring, and chromosome deletions such as 46,X,del(Xp). You may see Turner's syndrome written as 45,XO which is incorrect nomenclature (there is no "O" chromosome).

Case Conclusion You obtain chromosome analysis that shows 45,X karyotype. Follicle-stimulating hormone (FSH) is markedly elevated at 89 mIU/mL. You discuss management in terms of using growth hormone therapy to enhance growth and starting estrogen-replacement therapy to bring on secondary sexual changes and long-term prevention of osteoporosis. Lastly, you mention that conception, through in vitro fertilization (IVF) using donor eggs, is an option for her later in life.

Thumbnail: Sex Chromosomes

XXX females: no physical abnormalities; average IQ 10 to 20 points lower than that of controls; normal reproduction; 90% from a maternal nondisjunction in meiosis I

XYY males: normal appearance, taller than average; IQ 10 to 20 points lower than that of controls; tendency for emotional immaturity and impulsive behavior; result from nondisjunction in paternal meiosis II or postzygotic event

XXY (Klinefelter's syndrome) males: taller than average, breast development (gynecomastia), small testes, and infertility; additional X chromosome either paternally or maternally derived; generally of normal intelligence, but may have language learning disabilities

All trisomies (21, 18, 13, XXX, XXY) show maternal age effect; the paternally derived trisomies have not been shown to have an advancing age effect (nondisjunction during meiosis II)

Key Points

▸ Most common cause of primary amenorrhea.

▸ Short stature, congenital lymphedema, and ovarian dysgenesis are hallmarks of Turner syndrome.

▸ Growth hormone therapy, estrogen-replacement therapy, and r/o congenital heart disease are mainstays of management.

▸ No advanced maternal age effect, usually sporadic (low recurrence risk).

Questions

1. A 10-year-old girl has hemophilia A. She is as severely affected as her 13-year-old brother. This could be explained by which of the following?

   A. Homozygous for this X-linked recessive disorder
   B. Skewed X inactivation
   C. 45,X karyotyped female with hemophilia A
   D. X-autosome translocations
   E. All of the above

2. A newborn female with a prominent clitoris has been diagnosed with Turner's syndrome. Her karyotype is 45,X/46,XY. Which of the following would you recommend?

   A. Immediate removal of the gonads
   B. Prophylactic removal of the gonads after puberty
   C. Bilateral oophorectomy if an ovarian tumor develops
   D. Routine management for Turner's syndrome (same as for monosomy X)
   E. None of the above

3. The wide range of phenotypes for the various sex chromosome abnormalities can be explained at least in part by which of the following?

   A. Bias of ascertainment by studying only individuals that present with problems
   B. Imprinting effect due to parental origin of nondisjunction
   C. Data obtained prenatally may be different from data from postnatal ascertainment
   D. A and C are correct
   E. A and B are correct

HPI: PS calls your office with complaints of vaginal bleeding and lower abdominal cramping. She also noticed the presence of small grapelike tissue within the blood clots. In addition, she complains of terrible "morning sickness" for the last week. Currently, she is 9 weeks from her last menstrual period (LMP). Her medical history is unremarkable. This is her second pregnancy.

PE: Pulse 100, BP 120/80, temperature 37.1°C
Adult female in no acute distress. Head and neck unremarkable. No thyroid enlargement. Cardiopulmonary within normal limits. Abdomen is soft and nontender. Pelvic exam is notable for uterine size of 12 weeks' gestation and bilateral large adnexal masses. Minimal active bleeding through external cervical os.

Labs: β-hCG 1,000,602 mIU/mL, blood type A, Rh positive
Pelvic ultrasound shows her uterus is occupied by heterogenous material, with "snowstorm" appearance. Both ovaries are enlarged, containing several hypoechoic cysts.

Thought Questions

- What is the diagnosis?
- What is the clinical presentation and prognosis?
- What is the genetic mechanism involved?
- How is this condition treated?

Basic Science Review and Discussion

Hydatidiform Moles   Occasionally conception results in an abnormal pregnancy in which the placenta consists of a proliferation of a disorganized mass known as **hydatidiform mole** or **molar pregnancy,** which are classified as **complete** or **partial** based on their karyotype, gross morphology, and histopathology.

The most common presenting symptom in a molar pregnancy is vaginal bleeding. Other typical signs and symptoms include a uterine size larger than expected for dates due to the rapid proliferation of tissue, hCG levels higher than 100,000, large bilateral thecal lutein ovarian cysts, early presentation of preeclampsia, hyperthyroidism, and hyperemesis gravidarum. Many of these signs and symptoms are due to the **marked elevation of hCG.** Because of **early diagnosis due to the widespread use of US and quantitative hCG assay,** the diagnosis of hydatidiform mole is made usually in the first trimester and the classic signs and symptoms are seen less frequently. Once the diagnosis is suspected on clinical grounds, hCG levels, and sonography, care must be taken to exclude the medical complications that often coexist in the setting of a molar pregnancy. Once the medical status is stable, the treatment of choice is dilation and curettage (D&C) of the uterus for women who

wish to preserve their fertility. Eighty percent of molar pregnancies follow spontaneous resolution after D&C, but twenty percent will have persistent gestational trophoblastic disease (GTD). Four percent to six percent have metastatic disease and 16% local invasion. **Strict follow-up** with serial hCG measurements is necessary, along with **effective means of contraception** for 6 months after normalization (<2 mIU/mL) of hCG levels. This is because it would be difficult to differentiate between persistent GTD and a normal pregnancy. The risk of recurrence in future pregnancies is 1%.

Developmental Genetics of Molar Pregnancies   Complete hydatidiform moles have 46 chromosomes but are of exclusive paternal origin. A complete mole is caused by fertilization of an empty egg by two sperm or a single sperm that undergoes **endoreduplication.** The lethality observed in this condition is explained by the concept of **DNA-methylation imprinting,** which differentiates the maternal from the paternal set of chromosomes and regulates gene expression differentially.

In **partial moles,** the karyotype reveals the presence of 69 chromosomes (triploidy). Using DNA polymorphisms, it has been shown that 46 of these chromosomes are of paternal origin and the remaining 23 are of maternal origin. This **duplication of the normal paternal haploid** can be due to either fertilization of the egg by two sperm **(dispermy)** or duplication of the haploid set **(endoreduplication).** These fetuses are not compatible with life.

Observations in complete and partial moles indicate that paternally derived genes are essential in trophoblast development (there is no formation of fetal tissue in complete moles, which are only paternally derived) and maternally derived genes are necessary for early embryonic development.

Case Conclusion Before undergoing D&C, you obtain a chest x-ray and LFTs to exclude metastatic disease. PA had an uncomplicated D&C. She recovered promptly, with cessation of her nausea and vomiting and vaginal bleeding. Her hCG levels were monitored weekly until they were negative times three and then monthly for the next 6 months. She was placed on birth control pills during that time.

Thumbnail: Gene Dosage

Characteristics of Partial and Complete Moles

	Partial	Complete
Number of chromosomes	69	46
Paternal origin of chromosomes	23 maternal, 46 paternal	All paternal
Fetus present	Yes, but nonviable	No
Malignant potential	Very low	High

Key Points

▶ Paternally derived genes are essential for trophoblast development.

▶ Maternally derived genes are necessary for early embryonic development.

▶ DNA-methylation–mediated imprinting differentiates the maternal from the paternal set of chromosomes, regulates gene expression, and explains the early lethality seen in molar pregnancies.

Questions

1. Fetal demise with the presence of a large hydropic placenta was detected. The fetal karyotype revealed 69 chromosomes. What is the mechanism leading to this condition?

   A. Fertilization of a single ovum by two sperm
   B. Duplication of a haploid sperm chromosome set
   C. Duplication of a male-derived chromosome set and empty ovum
   D. Failure to undergo second meiotic division in the developing ova
   E. A and B are correct

2. Mature ovarian teratomas, or dermoid cysts, are one of the most common benign ovarian tumors, with a peak incidence in the second and third decades of life. What is the chromosomal complement of mature ovarian teratomas?

   A. 46,XX
   B. 46,XY
   C. 46,XX, all maternally derived
   D. 46,XX, all paternally derived
   E. 69 chromosomes: 23 maternally derived, 46 paternally derived

3. The hyperthyroid state that is occasionally seen in molar pregnancies can be explained by which of the following?

   A. Coincidence of two fairly common conditions in young women
   B. hCG has thyroid-stimulating activity; excessive hCG secretion may cause hyperthyroidism
   C. Suppression of serum TSH levels, due to increases in free thyroxine (T_4)
   D. High levels of hCG lead to an autoimmune state
   E. None of the above

HPI: EY is a 2-year-old boy who was referred to you by his pediatrician for seizures and developmental delay. You learn that as an infant, EY exhibited poor feeding, was hyperactive, and had trouble sleeping through the night. As he grew older, his developmental problems became more pronounced, with significant delays in learning how to sit and walk. He is still unable to speak (at this age, children should have a vocabulary of 50 words and should be using 2-word sentences). Six months ago, EY began having staring spells, which were eventually diagnosed as absence seizures. The parents are tired, frazzled, and very anxious for a diagnosis. Despite all that they have gone through, his parents added that EY is probably the happiest and most sociable of all their children.

PE: EY has a happy demeanor and laughs easily at trivial things in the office. His skin is much fairer than that of either parent. He has a smaller than average head, deep-set eyes, and a wide mouth. His gait is wide and ataxic. The remainder of his exam shows no abnormalities.

Thought Questions

- What is the most likely diagnosis?

- What is the inheritance pattern of this disease?

- What are some of the possible genetic defects causing this disease?

- What tests and/or studies would you order to confirm your diagnosis?

Basic Science Review and Discussion

Syndrome Description Angelman's and Prader-Willi syndromes are genetically inherited disorders. These distinct diseases result from a deletion on the long arm of chromosome 15 (15q11-q13). **Angelman's syndrome** occurs when this **deletion is inherited from the mother** and **Prader-Willi syndrome** results when it is **inherited from the father.** Angelman's syndrome consists of physical, neurologic, and developmental symptoms including severe mental retardation, general developmental delay, uncoordinated gait, seizures, hyperactivity, and disrupted sleep pattern. These patients often exhibit hypopigmented skin, mild physical dysmorphia (microcephaly, deep-set eyes, large mouth), and a characteristically happy disposition associated with excessive laughter. In contrast, the hallmarks of Prader-Willi syndrome include mild to moderate mental retardation, decreased muscle tone, hypothalamic insufficiency manifesting as hyperphagia and obesity, genital hypoplasia, incomplete or delayed puberty, and short stature.

Genomic Imprinting Considering that the Angelman and Prader-Willi syndromes derive from deletions of the same chromosomal region, these syndromes have a surprisingly dissimilar constellation of symptoms. This difference in phenotype can be attributed to the concept of genomic imprinting. Genomic imprinting is the differential expression of genes depending on its chromosome of origin (either maternal or paternal). In other words, the expression of certain chromosomes—whether the genes will be turned "on" or "off"—depends on whether the chromosome is inherited from the mother or the father. This process is controlled by an imprinting center within the chromosome and is likely to be due to differences in DNA-methylation (which involves adding methyl [CH_3] groups to nucleotides and thus inactivating the DNA). There are genes that are expressed only on the maternally derived chromosome, with the corresponding genes on the paternal chromosome remaining transcriptionally silent (and vice versa). Thus, deletion of part of a single chromosome will cause the loss of different sets of expressed genes, depending on whether the chromosome was from the mother or the father. This explains the differences between the Angelman and Prader-Willi syndromes: Angelman's syndrome is caused by deletion of the 15q11-q13 region on the maternal chromosome, and Prader-Willi is caused by deletion of the 15q11-q13 region on the paternal chromosome.

Genetic Defects There are several causes for the Angelman and Prader-Willi syndromes, including mutations and uniparental disomy. **Mutations** are any changes in the DNA code, such as substitutions and deletions, that may eventually lead to a change in the protein end product. In many children with these syndromes, large deletions within the 15q11-q13 region have been found, as well as small microdeletions that are present either within the imprinting center or in other genes in the region. In other cases, children can be affected through **uniparental disomy** in which they inherit both copies of their chromosome 15 from one parent. If both copies are from the father, the child will have Angelman's syndrome (consider this as the loss of the maternal chromosome), and if both copies are from the mother, the child will have Prader-Willi syndrome (consider this as the loss of the paternal chromosome).

Case Conclusion   From EY's history and physical exam, you suspect Angelman's syndrome. You perform a FISH analysis using a fluorescent probe specific for the 15q11-q13 region. You find that only one of the probes lights up, demonstrating that there is a large deletion in the maternal region and confirming your diagnosis.

EY's parents are relieved at finally having a diagnosis after years of blaming themselves for their son's condition. His seizures have been brought under control with medications and his sleeping pattern has improved as he has grown older. Although EY is still unable to speak, he is beginning to learn sign language in a specialized school at age 5 years. With the help of physical therapy, he is also learning to feed himself and to become toilet trained.

Thumbnail: Genomic Imprinting

Uniparental Disomy

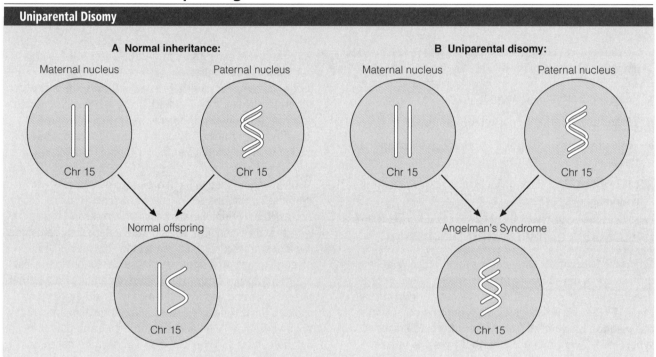

Key Points

- Genetic defect on maternal chromosome 15 results in Angelman's syndrome. Defect on paternal chromosome 15 results in Prader-Willi syndrome.
- The hallmarks of Angelman's syndrome include (1) mental retardation, (2) uncoordinated gait, (3) seizures, (4) absent speech, and (5) an excessively happy demeanor.

- The hallmarks of Prader-Willi syndrome include (1) mental retardation, (2) hyperphagia and obesity, (3) hypogonadism, and (4) short stature.
- Genetic imprinting is the differential expression of genes depending on their parental origin.
- Genetic defect can be due to large deletions, microdeletions, or uniparental disomy.

Questions

1. Assume that EY is able to reproduce. Hypothetically, what are the chances that his children will have Angelman's syndrome?

   A. 100%

   B. 66%

   C. 50%

   D. 25%

   E. 0%

2. Assuming EY's mutation is inheritable and is passed on for several generations to both male and female children, what inheritance pattern would the resulting pedigree (for Angelman's syndrome) mimic?

   A. AR

   B. AD

   C. X-linked recessive

   D. Mitochondrial inheritance

   E. None of the above

3. The differences in Angelman's and Prader-Willi syndromes are caused by differences in genetic imprinting flaws. Which of the following disorders are also caused by defects in genetic imprinting?

   A. Duchenne's muscular dystrophy

   B. Beckwith-Wiedemann syndrome

   C. NF

   D. CF

   E. Sickle-cell anemia

HPI: A 26-year-old man is seen in the ED for fever and shortness of breath. The patient has had 1 week of fever, non-productive cough, and progressive dyspnea. He has had two episodes of pneumonia within the past year, both times successfully treated with antibiotics. He also notes a 15-pound weight loss over the past year despite a healthy appetite. The patient has a history of IV heroin abuse but has been clean for the past 4 years. He currently works as a drug abuse counselor and is the single parent of a 4-year-old girl. He denies any other medical problems or any significant family history of medical diseases.

PE: T 39.5°C, BP 132/85, P 99 beats/min, RR 32 breaths/min, O_2 Sat 89%
The patient is sitting anxiously on the exam bed and is a lethargic and cachexic-appearing man in obvious respiratory distress. HEENT exam shows moderate anterior cervical chain lymphadenopathy. Lung exam reveals bilateral coarse breath sounds. He is tachypneic and using his accessory muscles of respiration.

Labs: WBC 9.1, chest x-ray bilateral interstitial opacities, CD4 81/μL, induced sputum Gram/silver stain and culture pending.

Thought Questions

- What is the likely cause for the patient's respiratory symptoms?

- What is the treatment for his respiratory tract infection?

- What is the underlying cause of the patient's immunodeficiency?

- How does this disease infect and replicate in the human body?

Basic Science Review and Discussion

Human immunodeficiency virus (HIV) is a retrovirus transmitted through either sexual contact, exposure to infected blood, or vertically from mother to child. After entry into the body, the virus infects CD4+ cells including macrophages during early infection and helper T-cells late in infection. **Acute infection** is marked by a rapid rise in the amount of virus found in the serum and a mononucleosis-like illness (fatigue, fever, headache, and muscle ache) in greater than half of all patients. The acute phase is followed by a reduction of plasma viremia to low steady-state levels correlated with a prolonged lack of symptoms clinically. Over time, the immune system wears down from its continuous struggle with HIV and there is a gradual decline in the number of helper T-cells. When the number of CD4+ cell count declines to less than 200/μL, immunocompromised patients become susceptible to various infections including ***Pneumocystis carinii* pneumonia (PCP)**. Symptoms of this infection include fever, progressive dyspnea, nonproductive cough, fatigue, chest pain, chills, and weight loss.

Specific tests for HIV include enzyme-linked immunosorbent assay (ELISA) test for the presence of HIV antibodies. A positive result can then be confirmed with a Western blot analysis, in which viral proteins are separated on a gel with electrophoresis, transferred to nitrocellulose filters, and incubated with serum from the patient. If the serum contains HIV-1 antibodies, they will bind to the antigens on the filters and be subsequently visualized. Other measures of an HIV infection include the CD4+ cell count (normally >800/μL) and HIV viral load measuring the amount of actively replicating HIV virus.

The diagnosis of PCP is commonly made by staining an induced sputum or bronchoalveolar lavage sample with either Giemsa or methenamine silver stain to detect cysts. Immunofluorescence study with monoclonal antibodies against *P. carinii* can also be used. Treatment is with trimethoprim-sulfamethoxazole (TMP-SMX) for 21 days and adjunctive therapy with corticosteroids.

Viral Genetics Retroviruses compose a family of **enveloped RNA viruses** that replicate by first using a reverse-transcriptase protein to produce DNA versions of their genome and subsequently integrate the DNA provirus into the host genome. This family of human retroviruses includes both the lentiviruses (HIV-1 and HIV-2) and the onc viruses (human T-cell lymphoma/leukemia viruses [HTLV-1 and HTLV-2]). HIV is composed of an outer lipid bilayer (envelope) and an inner nucleocapsid core containing two molecules of single-stranded RNA and other viral proteins such as reverse transcriptase and integrase. The HIV genome encodes for three genes common to all retroviruses *(gag, env, pol)*, as well as six accessory genes *(vif, vpr, vpu, rev, tat,* and *nef)* that are important in the regulation of HIV replication and infectivity. The life cycle of HIV includes an early infectious phase composed of viral attachment, entry, reverse transcription, and integration. This is followed by a much longer second phase, involving transcription of the viral genes and production of new viral particles.

Cellular entry is mediated by the binding of the gp120 viral envelope protein to the host cell CD4 receptor. This is followed by the **fusion** of the viral envelope with the cell membrane and the release of the viral RNA and enzymes into the cell. In the cytoplasm, the reverse transcriptase makes double-stranded DNA from the viral genomic RNA. After the DNA-protein complex is transported into the nucleus, the viral DNA genome (provirus) is incorporated into the host chromosome with the enzyme **integrase.**

When integration is complete, the viral genome becomes a permanent part of the host cell chromosome and will replicate along with the cell. The integrated HIV genome can either remain transcriptionally silent or become activated to produce viral progeny. The level of virus formed is mediated by several external factors including the presence of another infection, inflammatory cytokines, and host cellular activation. Production of new HIV-1 particles begins with the transcription of viral mRNA by host RNA polymerase II enzyme. The early protein products (HIV Tat, Rev, Nef) serve to control the process of virus production, and the late transcription products from the *gag, pol, env, vpu, vpr,* and *vif* genes are spliced by the viral protease into structural and late proteins. After assembly, the mature viral particles bud from the cell surface, completing the viral life cycle (Figure 33-1).

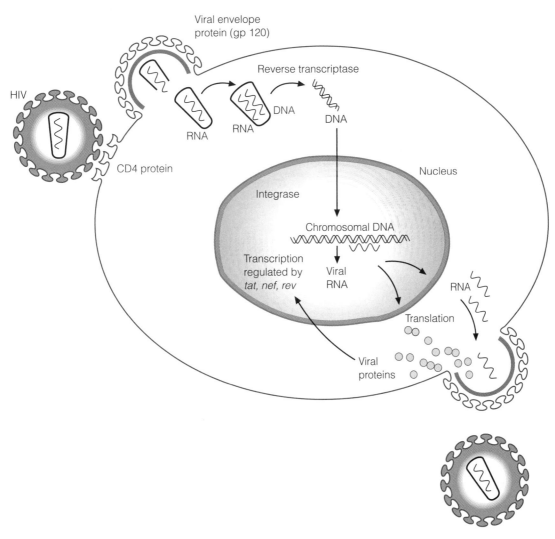

Figure 33-1 HIV life cycle.

Case Conclusion   The patient is found to have anti-HIV antibodies with an ELISA test that is confirmed with a Western blot. He has a viral load of 39,000 copies/mL. The induced sputum sample is stained with methenamine silver, which reveals cysts—confirming the clinical suspicion of PCP infection. The patient's respiratory symptoms gradually improve with treatment with TMP-SMX and corticosteroids. After discharge from the hospital, the patient is seen by his primary care physician and is started on antiviral therapy.

Thumbnail: Viral Genetics

Life Cycle of HIV

Step	Description
Attachment/entry	Viral envelope protein (gp120) binds to the host cell CD4 receptor and co-receptors, leading to the fusion of virus envelope with host cell membrane
Reverse transcription	Viral enzyme reverse transcriptase creates a DNA copy of the HIV RNA genome
Integration	Viral DNA is integrated into the host genome by the enzyme integrase
Transcription/translation	HIV mRNA/proteins are transcribed/translated from the integrated viral DNA by the host cell machinery
Assembly	Viral proteins are cleaved by the enzyme protease into their functional forms and packaged into progeny virus

HIV Genes and Their Products/Function

Gene	Gene products
gag	Four nucleocapsid proteins: p7, p9, p17, and p24
pol	Four enzymes: reverse transcriptase, integrase, ribonuclease H (RNase H), and protease
env	Two envelope proteins: gp41 and gp120
vif	Important in the production of infectious HIV particles
vpr	Regulates the import of viral DNA into the nucleus and aids in HIV pathogenesis
vpu	Mediates the degradation of the CD4 receptor and enhances the release of new virions
rev	Regulates HIV mRNA expression
tat	Regulates HIV mRNA expression
nef	Enhances viral replication/infectivity, and CD4/class I MHC down-regulation

Key Points

▶ HIV is transmitted by blood exposure, sexual contact, and vertically (during pregnancy).

▶ HIV infects CD4$^+$ macrophages (early) and helper T-cells (late).

▶ Acute HIV syndrome is the flu-like illness (fever, contact, fatigue, muscle ache, lymphadenopathy) frequently seen in the early stage of HIV infection.

Questions

1. HIV viral particles are blood borne and when transmitted are able to enter host cells and replicate. This process is dependent on a variety of HIV and host molecular machinery. Which of the following is not part of a mature HIV virus but is produced only after HIV has entered a host cell?

   A. HIV RNA
   B. Reverse transcriptase
   C. Viral envelope (gp120)
   D. HIV DNA
   E. Integrase

2. A number of pharmaceuticals are being used to treat HIV infections. Among these are protease inhibitors, which when used in combination therapy can bring the HIV viral load down precipitously. A protease inhibitor blocks which part of the HIV life cycle?

   A. Assembly
   B. Integration
   C. Reverse transcription
   D. Attachment
   E. Translation

3. In a laboratory studying viral genetics, fluorescence-tagged amino acids and nucleotides thymine and uracil are introduced into CD4$^+$ cells stably infected with HIV (with an integrated provirus). As new viruses bud from these cells, they are isolated and their fluorescence measured. Which of the following will be found to be fluorescence tagged in the new viral particles?

   A. Uracil only
   B. Uracil and thymine
   C. Thymine only
   D. Uracil and amino acids
   E. Uracil, thymine, and amino acids

HPI: LA is a 3-month-old African-American male infant who is brought in to the clinic for a follow-up exam. There has been concern that LA is falling off the growth curve.

PE: He is somewhat jaundiced. Other significant findings include frontal bossing and hepatosplenomegaly.

Labs: Reveal a severe microcytic anemia and a low reticulocyte count. The peripheral smear was reviewed and showed marked anisocytosis, poikilocytosis, hypochromia, and many target cells. A Hgb electrophoresis was ordered and Hgb A was found to be markedly decreased. Hgb F was found to comprise approximately 75% of the total Hgb.

Thought Questions

■ What are thalassemias? What are the different types? Which thalassemia is this child likely to have?

■ What are the genetic defects responsible for the different thalassemias?

■ What biochemical processes in the production of the β-globin protein are affected?

■ What is the clinical phenotype of β-thalassemia?

Basic Science Review and Discussion

β-Thalassemia Thalassemias are a set of **hereditary hemolytic anemias** that are caused by mutations that result in the **reduction in the synthesis of either the α or β chains** that make up the Hgb molecule. The reduction of a particular chain leads to the imbalance of globin chain synthesis and subsequently a distortion in the α/β ratio. As a result, **unpaired globin chains produce insoluble tetramers that precipitate** in the cell and cause damage to membranes. The RBCs are susceptible to premature RBC destruction by the reticuloendothelial system in the bone marrow, liver, and spleen.

In **β-thalassemia,** there is an **impairment of β-globin production** that leads to an excess of α chains. These disorders are typically **diagnosed several months after birth** because the presence of β-globin is only important postnatally when it would normally replace the γ-globin as the major non-α chain. There are multiple types of mutations that can lead to β-thalassemia. Almost any point mutation that causes a decrease in synthesis of mRNA or protein can cause this disease.

Transcription and Translation Let us first briefly review some basics on the flow of genetic information as it is transformed from DNA to RNA to protein. **Transcription** is the process of **creating an RNA** message from a DNA template. **Translation** is the **synthesis of protein** from RNA. Most genes are discontinuous, meaning that the primary RNA transcript contains **intervening noncoded sequences (introns)** that are split from the **coded message (exons)** to give the final RNA. **Small nuclear ribonucleoprotein particles (snRNPs)** mediate RNA splicing by binding to the primary RNA transcript and forming **spliceosomes.** There are multiple types of RNA: mRNA, ribosomal RNA (rRNA), transfer RNA (tRNA), and small nuclear RNA (snRNA).

Translation of the final mRNA into protein involves the coordinated activity of more than 100 other molecules. There are three phases in protein synthesis: **initiation, elongation,** and **termination.** A 40S ribosomal subunit containing the initiator tRNA, which always carries a methionine, and other initiation factors binds to the 5' cap binding region on the mRNA and scans along the mRNA until it discovers the first AUG or more rarely a GUG codon. The initiation factors dissociate and a 60S subunit then joins the 40S subunit to form an 80S initiation complex that is able to continue the elongation process. Elongation occurs in the 5' to 3' direction in a **GTP-dependent process** until a termination sequence is encountered. Specific release factors, which recognize the termination codons, mediate the hydrolysis of the bond between the elongating polypeptide and tRNA.

β-Thalassemia In β-thalassemia, three main types of mutations lead to a reduction of β-globin mRNA. These are mutations that affect the promoter region, cap binding, and RNA splicing. Abnormalities in RNA splicing account for the majority of β-thalassemia cases with defective mRNA synthesis. Splicing defects are placed into three categories: splice junction mutations, intron mutations, and exon mutations. Splice junction mutations are mutations at either the 5' donor or the 3' acceptor splice junctions or in the consensus sequences surrounding the junctions and as a consequence lead to a complete loss of normal splicing. Intron mutations can activate cryptic splice sites, and these alternative splice sites compete with the normal sites. Mutations in exons can also affect RNA splicing by activating cryptic splice sites. Other defects seen are those that lead to frameshifts or nonsense mutations. These types of errors result in nonfunctional mRNA that cannot direct the synthesis of a complete polypeptide because of an early stop codon and consequently truncated and unstable globin molecules. Deletions, the last type of mutation to mention, however, are an infrequent cause of β-thalassemia.

There are two genes that encode for β-globin, and the location of the gene mutation determines the phenotype. The condition where β-globin production is absent is called β-thalassemia. β⁺-thalassemia is when β-chain synthesis is reduced. And finally, **thalassemia trait** is when one gene is normal and the other gene contains a mutation. Individuals with homozygous β-thalassemia do not present until 2 to 3 months after birth. It is characterized by increasing pallor associated with anemia. A blood smear typically shows

marked **anisocytosis, poikilocytosis,** and **hypochromia** and many **target cells.** Sometimes a slight leukocytosis and thrombocytosis is present secondary to bone marrow stimulation. The Hgb electrophoresis shows a marked decrease in Hgb A ($\alpha_2\beta_2$) and an increase in both Hgb A$_2$ ($\alpha_2\delta_2$) and F ($\alpha_2\gamma_2$). These patients require lifelong transfusion and iron chelation therapy. Those who do not receive transfusion treatment can have growth retardation and skeletal deformities caused by expansion of the bone marrow cavities. Individuals who are heterozygous for β-thalassemia are generally clinically well with only mild anemia and a slight reticulocytosis. Treatment is not necessary for these individuals.

Case Conclusion　LA requires a transfusion for his severe anemia. He is referred to a pediatric hematologist, who manages his transfusion and chelation therapy with desferrioxamine (to prevent iron overload with all the transfusions). There is discussion with his parents that with the regular transfusions he is receiving, he may need a splenectomy when he is older, at approximately age 6 to 8 years. The possibility of bone marrow transplant is also mentioned, but there are considerable risks with graft versus host disease. The hopes are that scientists will be able to develop a gene therapy for β-thalassemia, in which the β-globin gene can be inserted into patients so they can begin making their own β-globin.

Thumbnail: Gene Transcription and Translation

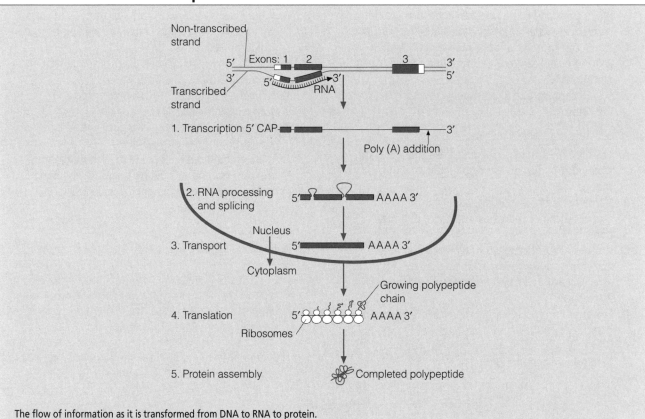

The flow of information as it is transformed from DNA to RNA to protein.

Key Points

▶ **Transcription** is creating RNA from a DNA template, and **translation** is converting the RNA message into a polypeptide.

▶ DNA, RNA, and protein synthesis all occur in the 5' to 3' direction.

▶ RNA processing involves capping the 5' end with 7-methylguanylate, splicing out introns from the primary mRNA transcripts (a process dependent on snRNPs), and polyadenylation of the 3' end by approximately 200 "A"s. This final capped and tailed transcript is the mRNA and is transported out of the nucleus for translation.

▶ Protein synthesis occurs in three basic steps: initiation, elongation, and termination. ATP is necessary for tRNA charging at the time of initiation to identification of the AUG start site, and GTP is necessary for elongation of the polypeptide and termination of this process.

▶ In β-thalassemia, there is impaired β-globin production, leading to a distortion in the α/β ratio, resulting in insoluble tetramers that precipitate in cells. This causes cell membrane damage and RBC destruction by the reticuloendothelial system.

▶ β-Thalassemia is caused mainly by splicing defects.

Questions

1. Genes are codes that specify the kinds of proteins that a cell should make. However, DNA itself does not function as a direct template for protein synthesis. Instead, RNA serves this role. Which of the following is true about RNA transcripts in human cells?

   A. Binding of the 5' cap by initiation factors occurs in the nucleus and is the first step in protein synthesis.

   B. Formation of spliceosomes is mediated by snRNPs.

   C. The 5' cap contains a formylmethionyl-tRNA.

   D. Splicing errors can result in nonsense or frameshift mutations.

   E. RNA 5' capping and 3' polyadenylation occurs in the cytosol.

2. Which statement about mutations is true?

   A. Missense mutations are often a base change at the third position but do not result in an amino acid change.

   B. Nonsense mutations are associated with more severe outcomes than missense and silent mutations.

   C. Nonsense mutations lead to a misreading of all nucleotides downstream of the mutation and usually result in a truncated protein from an early stop codon.

   D. Missense mutations lead to more severe outcomes than silent and frameshift mutations.

   E. Silent mutations lead to more severe outcomes than nonsense mutations.

3. Prokaryotes and eukaryotes share many similarities in transcriptions and translation. However, focusing on their differences allows pharmaceutical companies to find ways to target only microbes for new antibiotics. In eukaryotes, which of the following statements is true regarding protein synthesis?

   A. It begins with the AUG start site that is surrounded by a purine-rich region known as the Shine-Dalgarno sequence.

   B. It starts when the 30S and 50S ribosomal subunits bind the 5' cap of the mRNA.

   C. It involves an initiator tRNA that encodes N-formylmethionine (fMet).

   D. It requires GTP for tRNA charging and ATP for elongation of the polypeptide.

   E. It is terminated by release factors that recognize the stop codons and the hydrolysis of the bond between tRNA and the polypeptide in a GTP-dependent manner.

> **HPI:** TK is an 18-month-old male brought to the pediatrics clinic for his fifth bout of diarrhea. This is the first time you have seen TK. His mother has always been concerned that TK gets sick easily. However, his other doctors always blamed it on the day care center TK is at 6 days a week. The prenatal course, labor, and delivery of TK were routine. When he was 7 months, he started getting frequent infections, mainly GI, leading to diarrhea. Initially, this was attributed to his diet but did not improve despite all the nutritionist's recommendations. TK has also been seen for ear infections and colds and has had two short-stay hospitalizations. One hospitalization was for dehydration from severe diarrhea, and the other for pneumonia. Upon further discussion, you learn that the mother and her sisters all are healthy. However, she has a male cousin who is always sick and receives repeated shots for treatment.

Thought Questions

- What is agammaglobulinemia? What are the signs and symptoms?

- What is the defect causing this disease?

- Describe the structure of an immunoglobulin. What is unique about the genetics of immunoglobulins?

Basic Science Review and Discussion

X-linked Agammaglobulinemia X-linked agammaglobulinemia is a primary immunodeficiency that affects only males and is characterized by an absence of or a significant decrease in the amount of immunoglobulins synthesized. It occurs at a frequency of approximately 1 in 10,000. The defect has been localized to the central region of the long arm of the X chromosome, where a tyrosine kinase, BtK, is encoded. Although the details in the pathophysiology of this disease are still unclear, it is known that BtK is necessary for the maturation of pre-B-lymphocytes to mature B-lymphocytes. Typically, the sequence of B-cell differentiation occurs as follows: Stem cells in the bone marrow differentiate into pre-B-lymphocytes, and pre-B-lymphocytes mature into B-lymphocytes. When a mature B-lymphocyte is activated by binding a specific antigen it can differentiate into an antibody secreting plasma cell. In this disease, there is an absence of mature B-lymphocytes and plasma cells, and therefore, the body is unable to produce antibodies.

Only male individuals are affected by the X-linked form of agammaglobulinemia. Males typically present with early development of **serious pyogenic or viral infections.** They can present as early as 6 to 9 months of age, when maternal immunoglobulins have been degraded. The illnesses that affect these individuals are those that require **humoral immunity.** These individuals have an intact **cellular immunity** response, as evidenced by the presence of normal functioning T-cells. Common illnesses to which they are susceptible are those that occur at or near the surface of mucous membranes such as otitis, sinusitis, bronchitis, conjunctivitis, rhinitis, and gastroenteritis. Occasionally,

individuals are afflicted with osteomyelitis, meningitis, and sepsis. The most common pathogens seen in this disease are *Pneumococcus, Streptococcus, Staphylococcus,* and *Haemophilus influenzae.* Viruses can also cause disease, especially upper respiratory tract infections and gastroenteritis.

Tests used to confirm diagnosis include blood tests to evaluate serum immunoglobulin levels. A serum immunoelectrophoresis measures the presence of immunoglobulins and is able to delineate different types and whether they are polyclonal or monoclonal. A quantitative immunoglobulin analysis is used to quantitate the levels of each type of immunoglobulin present in a sample. In agammaglobulinemia, immunoglobulin G (IgG) levels are less than 200 mg/dL, and IgA, IgD, IgE, and IgM are almost not measurable. Additional tests include genetic studies to evaluate for a defect in the BtK gene. Of note, a CBC count on affected individuals is usually within the normal reference range. However, fractionation into the different cell components would reveal an absence in B-cells while the T-cell count is within the normal range. This is consistent with an intact cellular immunity response. Also, these individuals lack tonsils and adenoid tissue. Histologic examination of lymphoid tissue reveals an absence of germinal centers.

There is no cure for this disease. The goal of treatments is to replenish the body levels of immunoglobulins, and individuals receive regular treatments with IV immune globulin (IVIG). It is also important to treat infections aggressively with the appropriate antibiotics. The prognosis for these individuals is good if they are diagnosed early and receive regular treatments with immunoglobins and are aggressively treated for infections. These affected males are able to live a relatively normal life. However, they do have a shortened life span, secondary to chronic disease.

Immunoglobulin Structure Antibodies exist in two forms: membrane bound and secreted. Immunoglobulin molecules are composed of four polypeptide chains. There are two identical heavy chains and two identical light chains, and these are held together by disulfide bonds. The heavy chains are subdivided into five classes or isotypes, α, ϵ, δ, γ, and μ, corresponding to IgA, IgE, IgD, IgG, and IgM, respectively. The light chains are divided into two types, κ and λ. The antibody produced by a single B-cell will contain one type of heavy chain and one type of light chain. Each heavy and light chain has two segments, a constant (C) region and a variable (V) region. The constant region is located near the C-terminus and contains the sequences that define the isotype. The variable region is located at the amino-terminal, and the amino acid sequences here are highly varied between different immunoglobulins. The V regions of the heavy and light chains together define the specificity of antigen binding.

Immunoglobulin Genetics   The genetics of immunoglobulins is quite unique because they have the ability to undergo somatic rearrangement, allowing the finite genes defined by the germline to undergo rearrangements and generate an infinite number of different immunoglobulins. This ability to form a vast variety of antibodies is important for individuals to protect themselves from infectious organisms, toxic agents, and tumor cells. The heavy and light chains are encoded by multiple segments that are widely separated over three unlinked chromosomes. The light-chain V-region domain is encoded by a V and joining (J) segment. The heavy-chain V region is encoded by three gene segments, the V, J, and a diversity (D) segment. During B-cell differentiation, the DNA sequences for immunoglobulins under somatic rearrangement. In light chains, a single V and a single J come together with loss of the intervening segment, and together they form a complete variable region. Similarly, in the heavy chains, a single D and J segment combine, and then they are juxtaposed with a V segment, to form a complete variable region of the heavy chain. Junctional diversity also adds to antibody diversity. This is created by the imprecise joining of segments when there is a random insertion of nucleotides not encoded by the germline between the recombining V, D, and J segments. Furthermore, additional diversity of the variable regions is obtained through somatic point mutations within the variable region of genes. The final rearranged sequence is then transcribed with removal of any intervening sequences by RNA splicing, resulting in a mature RNA transcript. The transcript then undergoes translation and processing to form the final antibody product.

Case Conclusion   You suspect that TK has X-linked agammaglobulinemia. A serum immunoglobulin electrophoresis supports your suspicion and further genetic work-up confirms this diagnosis. TK is started on IVIG, and the frequency of his infections decreases. Based on the counseling that TK's mother obtained, she decides not to have more children. Ten years later, TK is still doing relatively well. He continues to receive regular infusions of immunoglobulins. Occasionally, he is hospitalized for a more severe infection requiring IV antibiotics. But overall, he is able to live a relatively normal life.

Thumbnail: Immunoglobulin Genetics

Immunoglobulin Class and Function

Ig type	% of total	Function class
IgA	13	Found in secretions; protects body surfaces and the GI tract
IgD	1	Function not clear
IgE	low	Involved in allergic reactions; protects against parasitic infections
IgG	80	Involved in fighting bacterial infections and neutralizing toxins; crosses the placenta and breast milk and provides passive immunity to fetus and infants
IgM	6	Antibody first formed in response to an antigen, best at fixing complement

Key Points

▶ Immunoglobulins:

1. There are five types of immunoglobulins, IgG, IgA, IgM, IgD, and IgE.

2. Immunoglobulins consist of a heavy and a light chain, and each chain is divided into a constant and a variable region.

3. Antibody diversity is obtained through somatic rearrangement of the germline genes encoding immunoglobulins, junctional diversity, somatic mutations within the genes encoding the variable region, and the various combinations made between the different heavy and light chains.

▶ X-linked Agammaglobulinemia:

1. An inherited primary immunodeficiency resulting from an absence of or a significant decrease in antibodies.

2. It is due to a defect in the ability of pre-B-cells to differentiate into mature B-cells and hence plasma cells. This defect has been linked to the tyrosine kinase BtK.

3. Affected individuals are susceptible to recurrent infections, especially those that affect mucosal surfaces.

4. Treatment includes repeated courses of IVIG administration and aggressive antibiotic therapy for infections.

Questions

1. It is estimated that the human genome can generate approximately 10^8 different antibodies. However, the genome is composed of only 3×10^9 bp of DNA. This vast diversity of antibodies is due in part to which of the following?

A. Homologous recombination
B. Translocation
C. Deletion
D. Point mutations
E. Duplication

2. X-linked agammaglobulinemia was first described in 1952 by Dr. Odgen Bruton, and this disease entity is also known an Bruton's agammaglobulinemia. Infants affected by this disease typically begin developing recurrent infections as early as 6 to 9 months, when a specific type of maternal immunoglobulin is eventually degraded. Which immunoglobulin is this?

A. IgA
B. IgD
C. IgE
D. IgG
E. IgM

HPI: ML is a 24-year-old woman who is G1 P0 at 29 weeks of gestation dated by a sure LMP who newly presents for prenatal care. She just recently moved from the refugee camps in Thailand. She has never had any formal medical care, and she has never been ill and has never had any surgical procedures.

PE: Unremarkable except for a fundal height measuring 33 cm. Prenatal labs were all normal except for a mild microcytic anemia and the absence of a rubella titer. That same day, ML also went for a routine obstetric US and findings were significant for ascites, pleural effusions, pericardial effusion, and pronounced skin thickening in the fetus consistent with fetal hydrops. Hgb electrophoresis was normal, but given the high suspicion for α-thalassemia, gene mapping studies were performed, which confirmed that ML has α-thalassemia trait.

Thought Questions

■ What is α-thalassemia?

■ What genetic defects are responsible for α-thalassemia?

■ How does the Hgb in this disease function differently?

Basic Science Review and Discussion

Hemoglobin is an oxygen-carrying molecule found in vertebrate RBCs, some invertebrates, and in the root nodule of legumes. It is a tetramer made of four polypeptide chains each containing a heme group. This heme group is an iron-containing pigment that combines with oxygen and gives Hgb the ability to transport oxygen. The predominant Hgb in adults is Hgb A, which consists of two α and two β subunits (denoted as α2,β2). Hgb is an allosteric protein with three special characteristics. First, the binding of O_2 to Hgb is cooperative, meaning that the binding of the first O_2 enhances the binding of additional O_2 on the same molecule. This property is reflected in the sigmoidal Hgb-oxygen binding curve. Secondly, H^+ and CO_2 promote the release of O_2 from Hgb in metabolically active tissues, and conversely, O_2 promotes the release of H^+ and CO_2 in the lungs. The relationship between O_2, H^+, and CO_2 is known as the Bohr effect. Third, the affinity of O_2 for Hgb is further regulated by 2,3-bisphosphoglycerate (BPG), a small highly anionic organic phosphate. BPG lowers the oxygen affinity of Hgb by approximately 26 times, which allows Hgb to unload oxygen in the tissue. BPG diminishes the affinity of oxygen to deoxygenated Hgb by binding to deoxy-Hgb at a central location where the four globin subunits interact.

Genetics of Hemoglobin   The normal Hgb molecule is made of two α-globin and two β-globin chains. There are, however, five other normal human Hgb molecules, each of which is also a tetrameric structure like Hgb A. These other Hgb molecules differ in subunit composition and their temporal expression during life. The α and α-like chains are encoded on chromosome 16. There are two α-globin genes, α1 and α2, which are present in tandem and each are expressed equally. The β and β-like chains are expressed on chromosome 11. Significant homology between β-globin and δ-globins exist, and they differ only in 10 out of 146 amino acids.

α-Thalassemia   α-Thalassemia is a genetic disease caused by a defect in α-globin synthesis, and it affects the formation of both fetal and adult Hgb. The most common cause for α-thalassemia is deletion. There are two identical α-chain genes on each chromosome 16, and the intron sequences surrounding these two genes are highly homologous, making misalignment, homologous pairing, and recombination between the two genes common events. Let us briefly review the concepts of deletions and duplications caused by recombination. Many genes have homologous sequences, placing them into groups of multigene families. If these genes are located in the same head-to-tail fashion in similar regions of a chromosome, they have a high probability of undergoing a crossover event, known as **homologous recombination.** This can occur between mispaired chromosomes or sister chromatids, resulting in unequal crossover events and subsequently gene deletion or duplication. Genetic diseases can also arise in recombination events in noncoding DNA regions.

With α-thalassemia, deletions or alterations of one, two, three, or four genes cause an increasingly severe phenotype. The most severe form of α-thalassemia causes fetal hydrops and is incompatible with life. These infants are pale, premature, and hydropic with severe anemia and splenomegaly. An Hgb electrophoresis would reveal no Hgb F and no Hgb A, and approximately 90% to 100% Hgb γ4, also referred to as Hgb Bart. Hgb H disease is due to the deletion of three α-globin genes, resulting in the accumulation of excess β chains in the RBC. Beta tetramers form, which are unstable and undergo oxidation. Membrane damage results, and these RBCs are susceptible to early clearance and destruction. These infants are born with anemia and the initial Hgb electrophoresis shows some Hgb

Bart and some Hgb H. Within the next few months, Hgb Bart disappears and the Hgb molecules detected are Hgb H and Hgb A. Peripheral smears show abnormal RBC morphology with hypochromia, microcytosis, target cells, and polychromasia. α-Thalassemia trait carries a milder phenotype with mainly a microcytic anemia and a normal Hgb electrophoresis. In this case, diagnosis is confirmed by gene mapping techniques.

Case Conclusion ML was seen by the perinatologist for counseling because it was clear that the prognosis of the fetus was poor. ML decided on expectant management of her pregnancy and declined any intervention. When ML was at 31 weeks of gestation, she presented to labor and delivery for decreased fetal movement and fetal heart tones could not be found. An ultrasound was performed immediately at bedside and confirmed a fetal demise.

Thumbnail: Protein Structure and Function

Homologous Recombination with α-Thalassemia

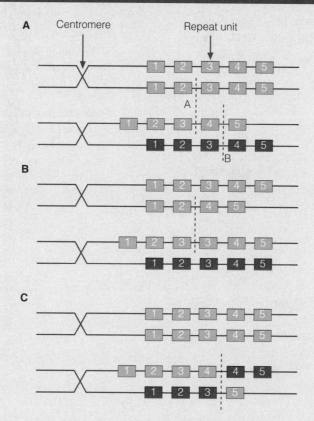

Unequal crossover occurs when the repetitive sequence region of a chromatid does not line up properly with the sister chromatid and therefore results in gene duplication or deletion.

Key Points

▶ Hgb is made of four polypeptide chains, each containing a heme group.

▶ Hgb is a model protein for the allosteric effect characterized by a sigmoidal oxygen-binding curve, the Bohr effect, and the regulation of O_2 affinity by BPG.

▶ BPG is a by-product of the glycolysis pathway and plays a critical role in the modulation of O_2 binding in Hgb.

▶ Gene deletions and duplications are often caused by the misalignment, homologous pairing, or recombination between two genes with homology.

Questions

1. In α-thalassemia, there is a defect in α-globin synthesis. As a consequence, one would expect which of the following?
   A. Precipitation of α-chain tetramers
   B. The carrier state to be clinically silent except for a mild microcytic anemia
   C. The genetic defect to be mainly due to single point mutations
   D. The affected individuals to be mostly of African or Mediterranean descent
   E. An absence of Hgb F

2. Ms. Li tells her sisters about her diagnosis and now her sisters want to be tested. Which of the following groups of tests include methods of gene mapping?
   A. Positional cloning, linkage analysis with RFLP, Western blot analysis
   B. Linkage analysis with RFLP, Western blot analysis, somatic cell hybridization
   C. Somatic cell hybridization, positional cloning, Western blot analysis
   D. Western blot analysis, FISH, somatic cell hybridization
   E. FISH, positional cloning, linkage analysis with RFLP

3. 2,3-BPG is known as a controller of oxygen transport in RBCs. These cells have high concentrations of 2,3-BPG, whereas most other cells only have trace amounts. Which is true regarding BPG?
   A. BPG binds strongly to fetal Hgb, so Hgb F has more affinity to oxygen than Hgb A.
   B. The action of BPG is to destabilize the Hgb complex, thereby decreasing its ability to bind oxygen.
   C. BPG is a by-product of the citric acid cycle.
   D. BPG lowers the O_2 affinity to Hgb by binding to the deoxy-Hgb but not the oxygenated form.
   E. BPG is considered a cofactor.

HPI: DR is a 4-year-old girl whose mother is concerned about speech and motor delays, as well as frequent infections. DR was the product of a full-term, uncomplicated pregnancy. Developmental milestones came at expected ages or a bit late. She walked at 16 months. Recently, DR's mother notes that her walk has become unsteadier. She also notices that her speech is slow and sometimes difficult to understand. During the past year, she has endured three bouts with pneumonia, more than five with otitis media, and one episode of skin herpes simplex virus (HSV) infection that required hospitalization.

PE: She is a happy little girl, nondysmorphic, growing at the fifth percentile for weight and height (parental height is in the fiftieth percentile). She has marked conjunctival telangiectasias that her mother points out appeared at age 3 years. Her gait is wide based and ataxic.

Labs: WBC 3.2, IgA *and* IgE markedly decreased, AFP 187 μg/L (normal range <3 μg/L)

Thought Questions

- What is the diagnosis? Can the diagnosis be confirmed?

- What is the natural history of this disorder?

- What are important management strategies for these patients?

- Are there health risks for the parents of this little girl?

Basic Science Review and Discussion:

Ataxia-Telangiectasia A-T is characterized by progressive cerebellar ataxia, choreoathetosis, oculocutaneous telangiectasias, serum and cellular immunodeficiencies, increased susceptibility to cancer, and hypersensitivity to ionizing radiation. The onset of neurological signs is between 1 and 3 years of age. By age 10 years, most patients with A-T are wheelchair bound. A small cerebellum is seen on MRI. The immunodeficiency leads to recurrent sinus-pulmonary infections. Reduced levels of IgA, IgE, and IgG2 are frequently found. Up to one third of patients with A-T will develop cancer, the majority being leukemia or lymphoma. As patients with A-T grow older, other cancer types may arise. Life expectancy for patients with A-T in the United States is

30 years, with pulmonary infections and malignancies being the major cause of death.

Increased chromosomal breakage and increased levels of AFP are found in most patients with A-T. These laboratory findings are helpful in establishing the diagnosis in patients who fit the clinical profile.

Genetics A-T is an AR disease caused by mutations of the A-T mutated (ATM) gene (chromosomal locus 11q22-q23). The large size of the **ATM** gene and the large number of possible mutations in patients with A-T greatly limit the utility of mutation analysis as a diagnostic tool, except in selected ethnic groups who have a small number of mutations that account for the majority of disease-causing mutant alleles.

DNA Repair and Inherited Cancer Several cancer syndromes occur as a result of germline mutations in DNA damage repair genes. These genes appear to have a rather passive role in cell growth, and their inactivation can result in an increased rate of mutations in cellular genes such as tumor suppressor genes and proto-oncogenes in affected cells. The ATM gene product is a kinase involved in mitogenic signaling, meiotic recombination, DNA repair, and cell cycle control.

Case Conclusion   You ordered chromosome analysis that showed a 46,XX karyotype with an increase in chromosomal breakage (10% of the metaphases analyzed). You started her on TMP-SMX (Septra) and acyclovir prophylaxis, as well as monthly IVIGs because of her immunosuppression. DR now uses sunscreen whenever outdoors. She also has begun physical therapy (PT) at school to help with her walk and avoid contractures. Frequent visits have been arranged for malignancy surveillance. Additionally, you spoke to DR's mother's primary care provider regarding her increased risk of breast cancer.

Thumbnail: DNA Repair

ATM, DNA Repair, and Cell Cycle

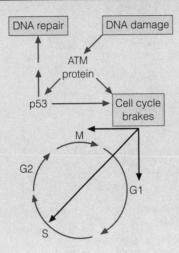

Key Points

- ▶ A-T: AR, cerebellar degeneration, oculocutaneous telangiectasias, increased risk of cancer, immuno-suppression

- ▶ Other DNA repair cancer syndromes: xeroderma pigmentosum, Bloom's syndrome, hereditary non-polyposis colon cancer (HNPCC)

Questions

1. Molecular studies on DR failed to identify any of the known disease-causing mutations in ataxia-telangectasia. If prenatal diagnosis is sought by this family, what modality is potentially possible to use?

   A. Not possible
   B. Second-trimester US
   C. AFP level in amniotic fluid
   D. Chromosomal breakable in amniocytes
   E. Linkage analysis

2. Costa Ricans, Mennonites, and other ethnic groups have an increased incidence of A-T and have few mutations that account for the majority of the disease-causing mutations for that specific group. These phenomena can be explained by which of the following?

   A. Increased rates of consanguinity
   B. Hardy-Weinberg principle
   C. Heterozygote advantage
   D. Founder effect
   E. Chance

HPI: LA is a 2-year-old female brought in for a routine physical exam. Her family had been living in England for the last year, so she has not received care from you since she was 1 year old. The mother reports that LA has overall been healthy over the last year. LA has been eating well and developing appropriately in size, motor, and language skills. The primary concern she reports to you is that LA seems to be increasingly cross-eyed.

PE: Remarkable for moderate strabismus, an inequality of pupil size, a slight difference in iris colors, and mild proptosis of the left eye. The red reflex of the left eye is notably absent.

Thought Questions

- What is retinoblastoma (Rb)? How is it obtained?

- What protein is responsible for this disease?

- Describe the normal cell cycle. What is the role of the Rb gene product?

Basic Science Review and Discussion

Rb is caused by a mutation in the **tumor suppressor** Rb gene, leading to a rare malignant tumor of the retina. It is found in approximately 1 in 20,000 births. Roughly 40% of cases are inherited, with an offspring obtaining a mutated allele through the germline, and the remaining 60% of cases occur sporadically. The signs of Rb include an absence of the **red reflex,** which typically is observed when light is directed at the retina. However, in the case of Rb, white is seen behind the pupils, which is also known as **leukocoria.** Other signs include strabismus or problems with eye movements, differences in pupil sizes, differences in iris colors, increased tearing, proptosis, nystagmus, and cataract formation. Most cases are diagnosed before the age of 5 years. The hereditary form is usually diagnosed earlier, with a mean age of 13 to 15 months, and the sporadic form is diagnosed at a mean age of 24 months. Treatment modalities include enucleation, external beam radiation, localized plaque radiation, photocoagulation, cryotherapy, and chemotherapy. The prognosis is overall good but generally depends on unilateral versus bilateral disease, extent of involvement, and age at diagnosis. One hundred years ago, the mortality rate from Rb was 100%. The death rate has since improved; in 1964, the mortality rate was 18%, and in 1990, it was less than 10%.

The Cell Cycle   To better understand the role of Rb, we will first review the general concepts of the cell cycle. The cell cycle is divided into four phases. **G1,** or **gap 1,** is the time when the cell prepares for DNA replication. Protein synthesis is significantly up-regulated at this time. In general, this is the portion of the cell cycle that varies from cell to cell, resulting in differences in doubling time between different cell types. On average, G1 lasts approximately 18 hours. **S phase** is the period when the cell undergoes **DNA replication,** and this typically lasts 20 hours. **G2,** or **gap 2,** is the period when the **cell prepares for cell division,** and this portion lasts roughly 3 hours. Lastly, **M phase,** or **mitosis,** is when the cell physically divides into two daughter cells and occurs over 1 hour. Cells that are not in the cell cycle are in **G0,** or **quiescent.** These cells may be temporarily out of the cell cycle, secondary to a negative stimulus such as lack of nutrients in the milieu or contact inhibition, which is a means of population control. Other cells are permanently out of the cell cycle because they have terminally differentiated, for example, neurons.

In general, three types of proteins interact with one another to orchestrate the progression through a cell cycle. **Cyclins** are proteins whose levels increase and decrease depending on the phase. There are different types of cyclins that are specific to each phase of the cell cycle or the transition of a phase. Cyclins serve a regulatory role to **cyclin-dependent kinases** (Cdks). The binding of a cyclin to its partner kinase allows the kinase to be activated. Cdks maintain a steady level throughout the cell cycle. Once bound to the appropriate cyclin, the kinase is able to phosphorylate downstream substrates, which include enzymes, structural proteins, and transcription factors. Cell cycle inhibitors also serve an integral role in the regulation of the cell cycle. These include tumor suppressors such as p53 and Rb and Cdk inhibitors like p27. Rb and p53 prevent cycle progression at the G1-S interface by interrupting transcription. p27 and other similar inhibitors, however, bind to active cyclin-Cdk complexes, inhibiting the kinase activity and the phosphorylation of downstream targets that are important for cell division.

Another important concept to understand is that **multiple checkpoints** exist within the cell cycle to prevent aberrant cell cycle progression. The first checkpoint is at the site of cell cycle entry from G0 to G1. This checkpoint ensures that the cell is ready for division with adequate resources available and an accommodating environment. The G1-S interface is the first checkpoint for DNA damage. It is the point that p53 and Rb govern. Other DNA checkpoints occur within the S phase and between the S phase and G2. These checkpoints monitor the presence of Okazaki's fragments during DNA replication, and a cell cannot proceed past the S phase until all the Okazaki fragments are gone. There is also a spindle checkpoint at the end of G2. It has been shown that cells that do not pass the checkpoints secondary to irreparable damage will undergo apoptosis.

Rb and p53 are guardians of the G1-S checkpoint. Rb has been shown to block cell cycle progression by binding to a transcription factor called **E2F** and thereby preventing the ability of E2F from binding promoters such as c-myc and c-fos. These proteins all regulate transcription of genes essential for proliferation. With one Rb allele absent, Rb can still be made from the unaffected allele, and Rb protein can still function to regulate the cell cycle. However, with two mutated Rb alleles, there is an absence of functioning Rb and cells with errors in the DNA replication are able to pass through these checkpoints, complete the cell cycle, and propagate their errors.

Case Conclusion   LA is diagnosed with Rb of the left eye. She is treated with localized plaque radiation therapy, but because of a lack of substantial response, she had to undergo an enucleation of the left eye. A genetic work-up determined that she had the sporadic form of Rb, and therefore, the enucleation was curative.

Thumbnail: Cell Cycle

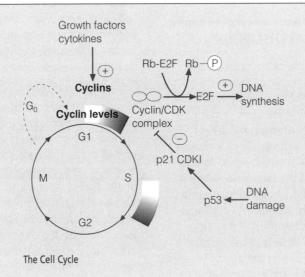

The Cell Cycle

Key Points

▶ The cell cycle consists of four phases: G1, S, G2, and M.

▶ Three types of proteins are important in the regulation of cell cycle progression. These are cyclins, Cdks, and inhibitors such as tumor suppressors or Cdk inhibitors.

▶ Multiple checkpoints exist within the cell cycle to prevent the propagation of errors.

▶ Rb is a rare malignant tumor of the retina resulting from a loss of function of the tumor suppressor Rb.

Questions

1. Some chemotherapeutic agents affect cells that are cycling and are specific to certain phases of the cycle. Tumor cells typically have a quicker doubling time than healthy tissues, making tumor cells more sensitive to chemotherapeutic agents. Which phase of the cell cycle is most variable and responsible for the differences in doubling time between different cell types?

   A. G0
   B. G1
   C. S
   D. G2
   E. M

2. There are many points of regulation involved in cell population control. These are all important to prevent the propagation of errors and the formation of malignancies. Which of the following is a form of regulation?

   A. The presence of the Okazaki fragments, preventing progression through S phase
   B. A decrease in p53, leading to a block in the G1-S interface
   C. Rb dissociation from E2F, resulting in a conformation change in E2F and the inability of E2F from functioning as a transcription factor
   D. p27 binding to Cdks, leading to activation of these kinases
   E. Cyclins binding to Cdks directly dephosphorylating downstream protein targets

Case 21

1 D
2 B
3 C
4 C

Case 22

1 B
2 B
3 D

Case 23

1 C
2 C
3 C
4 D

Case 24

1 C
2 D
3 A

Case 25

1 D
2 A
3 B

Case 26

1 D
2 E
3 C

Case 27

1 C
2 D
3 D

Case 28

1 B
2 B
3 E

Case 29

1 B
2 D
3 E

Case 30

1 E
2 B
3 D

Case 31

1 E
2 C
3 B

Case 32

1 E
2 E
3 B

Case 33

1 D
2 A
3 D

Case 34

1 B
2 B
3 E

Case 35

1 D
2 D

Case 36

1 E
2 E
3 D

Case 37

1 E
2 D

Case 38

1 B
2 A

Part III

Embryology

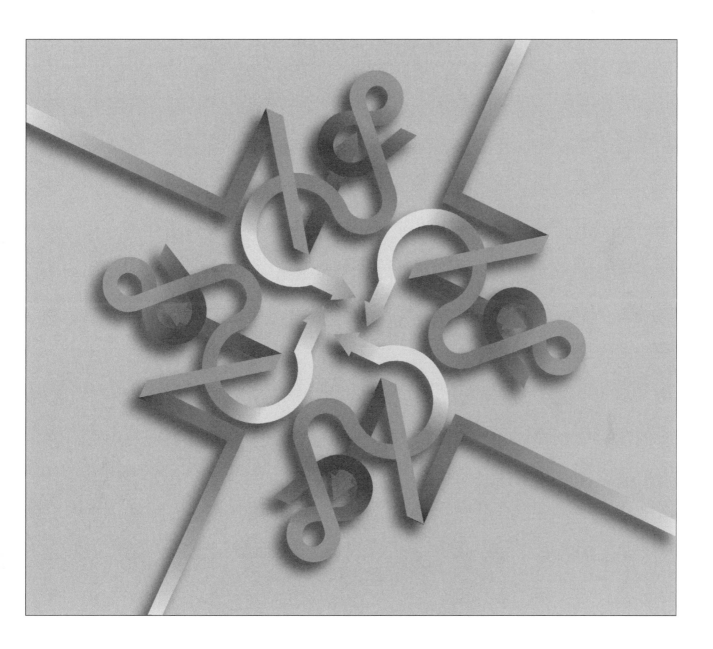

HPI: A 5-day-old baby girl is seen in the nursery by your team. She was found at birth to have bilateral congenital cataracts and low birth weight. She has also experienced poor feeding and a failure to thrive. The mother is a recent immigrant and received no prenatal care. She states that during the second month of the pregnancy, she had an unusual pinpoint, nonpruritic rash lasting for several days, which was preceded by flulike symptoms lasting about 1 week. The parents have two other children, now ages 3 and 5 years old, both of whom are healthy. They deny any significant family history of diseases.

PE: The infant appears lethargic and small. HEENT exam reveals mild microcephaly and bilateral cataracts. On cardiovascular exam, a grade 2/6 continuous machinery murmur is heard throughout the cardiac cycle. The remainder of her exam is normal.

Labs: Echocardiogram shows a patent ductus arteriosus (PDA). CT scan of the head reveals intracerebral calcifications.

Thought Questions

- What is the cause of the baby's defects?
- How is this disease transmitted?
- How is the timing of the mother's symptoms significant?
- What other infectious agents can cause birth defects?

Basic Science Review and Discussion

Syndrome Description Rubella is an enveloped RNA virus that is part of the togavirus family. It causes a mild infection in adults characterized by flulike symptoms for up to 1 week, followed by a fine, punctate, nonitchy rash lasting for 3 to 4 days. Infection of the fetus before 16 weeks of gestation can cause a wide range of congenital defects, whereas infection after the fifth month rarely leads to any morbidity. The most common defects include **sensorineural deafness, cataracts, cardiovascular defects** such as PDA and pulmonary artery stenosis, **CNS damage** leading to mental retardation, and **fetal growth restriction** (Figure 39-1). The advent of the rubella vaccination led to a dramatic decrease in the number of rubella-associated neonatal defects, but it is not effective for every individual, and even when successful, the duration of the immunity is often variable.

Diagnosis can be made by the detection of rubella-specific IgM antibodies in the infant, isolation of the virus from nasopharyngeal or urine specimens, or the persistence of rubella-specific IgG in the infant beyond the time expected due to just the passive transfer of maternal antibodies (usually after 8 to 12 months of age). There is no specific treatment for congenital rubella syndrome. Heart and eye defects can sometimes be corrected with surgery, and children with vision, hearing, or cognitive deficits can benefit from specialized education programs.

Organogenesis The period of **organogenesis** lasts from the third to the eighth week of gestation and is the time when most of the major organ systems are formed. For example, the embryonic eye first begins development on day 22, with the appearance of shallow grooves on either side of the forebrain. These grooves become the optic vesicle by the end of the fourth week and will induce the formation of the lens. By the end of the seventh week, the lens fibers are forming, as are the neural and pigment layers of the retina. During this critical period, the developing organs are very sensitive to both genetic and environmental insults. If a mother is infected with the rubella virus between the fourth and the seventh week of pregnancy, the resulting child will have a high risk of congenital cataracts. However, if infection is after the seventh week, the presence of a lens abnormality becomes rare. Similarly, cardiac malformations can occur with an infection before the first 12 weeks, and sensorineural deafness can occur if infection is before the first 16 weeks, but both defects are unusual with later infections.

Infectious Teratogens Rubella is one of several infectious organisms (including toxoplasmosis, rubella, CMV, herpes simplex virus, syphilis [ToRCHeS]) that can cause birth defects. Maternal infection with the protozoan *Toxoplasma gondii* can cause a flulike infection in the mother, as well as ocular (chorioretinitis, optic nerve atrophy), systemic (hepatosplenomegaly, jaundice), and CNS (microcephaly, mental retardation) manifestations in affected infants. **CMV** is a DNA herpesvirus that can cause a variety of CNS (microcephaly, mental retardation, hearing loss) and systemic (low birth weight, hepatosplenomegaly) symptoms. **HSV type 2** (HSV-2) is most likely to be transmitted during the delivery of the infant through the birth canal and can cause a syndrome of meningoencephalitis, seizures, and skin lesions. Intrauterine infection can be manifested by prematurity, low birth weight, microcephaly, chorioretinitis, and skin lesions. **Congenital syphilis** occurs when the spirochete is

Rubella syndrome

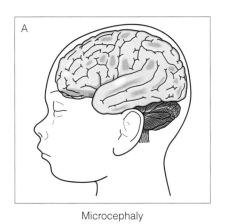

Microcephaly

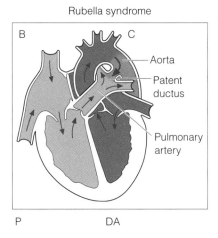

Aorta
Patent
ductus
Pulmonary
artery

P   DA

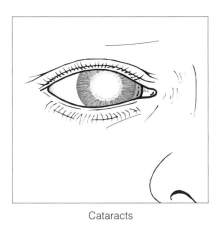

Cataracts

Figure 39-1 Teratogenic effects of rubella.

transmitted to the fetus and can result in a 40% fetal mortality rate, as well as a multiorgan infection causing bone or teeth deformities, rhinitis, rash on the palms and soles, mental retardation, and vision and hearing defects. In addition, many other infectious organisms have been found to have teratogenic effects, including HIV, varicellazoster, hepatitis B, *Parvovirus*, and *Chlamydia trachomatis*.

Case Conclusion   The infant is found to have rubella IgM antibodies, confirming the diagnosis of congenital rubella syndrome. She undergoes surgery to repair her heart defects, and after an extensive search, the parents are able to find an appropriate school for the visually and hearing impaired.

Thumbnail: Embryonic Development

Infectious Teratogens (ToRCHeS Organisms)	
Teratogen	**Symptoms**
Toxoplasmosis (*T. gondii*)	Ocular (chorioretinitis), hepatosplenomegaly, and CNS (mental retardation, hydrocephalus) malformations
Rubella	Sensorineural deafness, cataracts, cardiac abnormalities (PDA), CNS defects (microcephaly), and growth retardation
CMV	Microcephaly, hepatosplenomegaly, and blindness
HSV	Most infections at birth, but fetal infection can cause prematurity, growth retardation, mental retardation, and chorioretinitis
Syphilis (*Treponema pallidum*)	Multiorgan involvement including defects in bone formation, rash, rhinitis, mental retardation, deafness and vision loss

Key Points

▶ Rubella is an RNA virus that causes birth defects when fetal infection occurs before 16 weeks of gestation.

▶ Organogenesis lasts primarily from the third to the eighth week of gestation and is when the fetus is most sensitive to teratogens.

Questions

1. Infectious teratogens comprise a diverse class of organisms ranging from RNA viruses to DNA viruses to bacteria. Which of the following teratogenic syndromes is caused by a protozoan?

   A. Toxoplasmosis
   B. Rubella
   C. CMV
   D. HSV-2
   E. Syphilis

2. A newborn presents to your pediatric office with a history of poor feeding, failure to thrive, nasal discharge, and rash on the hands and feet. Which test would you order to definitively diagnose this infectious teratogen?

   A. Rubella IgG detection
   B. Rubella IgM detection
   C. HSV culture of blisters
   D. Urine culture for CMV
   E. Dark-field microscopy

3. A 30-year-old pregnant woman at 15 weeks of gestation is brought to the ED by a friend for fever, lethargy, and excessive sleepiness. The woman is known to be HIV positive, but the rest of her medical history is unobtainable. Physical exam is significant for cervical lymphadenopathy and altered mental status. Head CT reveals multiple ring-enhancing lesions and edema. Which of the following infectious teratogens are you most worried about?

   A. Toxoplasmosis
   B. Rubella
   C. CMV
   D. HSV-2
   E. Syphilis

HPI: You are called to evaluate a full-term male newborn with difficulty feeding and at risk of aspiration. The baby was recently delivered after an uncomplicated vaginal delivery. The mother reports that her pregnancy was uneventful, except for spotting during the second month. She states that there were no exposures to any medications, alcohol, drugs, or infections throughout the pregnancy. Review of a three-generation pedigree reveals that a paternal first-degree cousin was born with bilateral cleft lip.

PE: Full-term male infant in no acute distress. Height, weight, and head circumference are close to the fiftieth percentile. Examination of the face reveals a unilateral left cleft lip and a cleft palate. Systematic examination does not detect any other major or minor anomalies.

Thought Questions

- What are the steps involved in the formation of the face?

- What is the developmental error that causes this defect?

- What is the etiology of this malformation?

- How is this condition treated?

Basic Science Review and Discussion

Cleft lip and palate is one of the most common congenital anomalies, affecting 1 in 700 newborns. Cleft lip and palate can occur alone but more often arise together, and the condition **develops when the maxillary processes fail to grow medially and fuse with the frontonasal process.** The cleft anterior to the incisive foramen (primary) and that posterior to the foramen (secondary) define the anatomic delineation of cleft palate (Figure 40-1). The **primary palate** refers to that area that forms the upper lip, columella, maxillary alveolus, and the hard palate anterior to the incisive foramen. The **secondary palate** forms the soft and hard palate posterior to the incisive foramen. Between the fourth and eighth week of gestation, the primary palate formation is usually complete, and the formation of the secondary palate is completed between the eighth and twelfth weeks of gestation. **These distinctly different times for the development of the primary and secondary palates** form the basis for considering cleft lip with cleft palate and isolated cleft palate **different developmental deformities.**

Infants with isolated cleft lip rarely have feeding problems, whereas those with both cleft lip and palate or palate alone may require special nipples to help with feeding and avoid the risk of aspiration. Surgical repair is needed; the timing depends on the defect. For cleft lip, the "rule of 10s" applies—10 weeks, 10 pounds, Hgb level of 10. In cleft palate, surgical treatment occurs around 1 year, before speech develops. Subsequent surgical revisions may be required as the child grows.

Although the majority of cases of cleft lip with or without cleft palate occur as an isolated malformation, about **30% of cases occur as part of a syndrome** of birth defects that have cleft lip and/or palate as feature(s). A **precise diagnosis** is necessary before falling back on empiric risk figures for genetic counseling. The **risk of recurrence** in subsequently born children is 4% if one child has it, 4% if one parent has it, 17% if one parent and one child have it, and 9% if two children have it. **Isolated cleft lip and palate is of multifactorial etiology.**

Development of the Face   During the fourth and fifth weeks of gestation, the primitive pharynx is bounded laterally by the pharyngeal arches. Each arch is composed of a core of mesenchymal cells covered by ectoderm on the outside and endoderm on the inside. Neural crest cells migrate into the arches and are the source of the connective tissue. Each arch has an artery, a cartilage rod, a nerve, and a muscle component. Externally, the arches are separated by pharyngeal clefts, and, internally, they are separated by evaginations, or pouches. When the ectoderm of a cleft meets the endoderm of a pouch, a pharyngeal membrane is formed. The **development of the face, neck, and related structures is largely the result of transformation of the pharyngeal apparatus into adult structures.** Because of the complicated development of the face and palate, anomalies of these areas are common. Defects arise as a result of abnormalities in neural crest tissue migration or induction into the maxillary prominence of the first laryngeal arch (Figure 40-2, A and B)

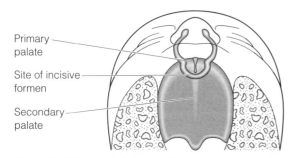

Primary palate

Site of incisive formen

Secondary palate

Figure 40-1 Bilateral cleft lip and cleft of the anterior palate.

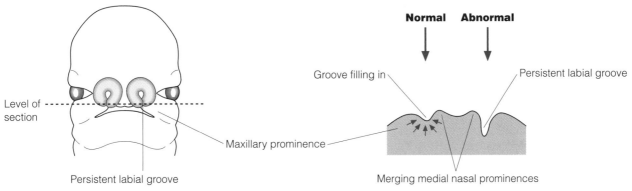

Figure 40-2 **A:** Development of the face. **B:** Formation of cleft lip.

Case Conclusion   The infant underwent his first surgical repair at age 3 months, followed by a second repair at 12 months. He has done well, is fully functional, and without limitation on his speech or swallowing. The parents decided to have another child 3 years later. A targeted fetal US at 18 weeks showed normal anatomy.

Thumbnail: Fetal Development

The Pharyngeal Apparatus				
Arch	**Nerve**	**Muscles**	**Skeletal structures**	**Ligaments**
First (mandibular)	Trigeminal (cranial nerve [CN] V)	Muscles of mastication Mylohyoid and anterior belly of digastric Tensor tympanic Tensor veli palatini	Malleus Incus	Anterior ligament of malleus Sphenomandibular ligament
Second (hyoid)	Facial (CN VII)	Muscles of facial expression Stapedius Stylohyoid Post belly of digastric	Stapes Styloid process Lesser cornu hyoid Upper part of body of hyoid bone	Stylohyoid ligament
Third	Glossopharyngeal (CN IX)	Stylopharyngeus	Greater cornu of hyoid Lower part of hyoid bone	
Fourth and sixth (the fifth arch is usually absent)	Superior laryngeal branch of the vagus (CN X) Recurrent laryngeal branch of the vagus (CN X)	Cricothyroid Levator veli palatini Constrictors of pharynx Intrinsic muscles of larynx Striated muscles of esophagus	Thyroid cartilage Cricoid cartilage Arytenoid cartilage Corniculate cartilage Cuneiforme cartilage	

Key Points

▶ Pharyngeal arches are made of a core of mesenchyme covered by ectoderm externally and endoderm internally.

▶ Externally, the arches are separated by clefts, and internally by pouches. The pharyngeal membranes are formed when the ectoderm of the clefts meets the endoderm of a pouch.

▶ Arches, clefts, pouches, and the pharyngeal membranes make up the pharyngeal apparatus.

▶ All clefts disappear, except the external acoustic meatus.

▶ All membranes disappear, except the first—the tympanic membrane.

Questions

1. DiGeorge's syndrome is characterized by aplasia of the thymus and parathyroid glands, distinct facial features, cleft palate, and conotruncal cardiac defects. The developmental error involves which of the following arches?

   A. First, second, and third pharyngeal arches

   B. First, third, and fourth pharyngeal arches

   C. Second and third pharyngeal arches

   D. Third and fourth arches

   E. Fourth, fifth, and sixth arches

2. Isolated cleft lip and palate is best characterized by which of the following?

   A. Single gene defect, developmental error between 8 to 12 weeks of gestation

   B. Chromosomal abnormality, developmental error between 4 and 8 weeks of gestation

   C. Alcohol exposure, developmental error between 4 and 6 weeks of gestation

   D. Cigarette smoking, developmental error between 5 and 8 weeks of gestation

   E. Multifactorial inheritance, developmental error between 5 and 8 weeks of gestation

3. Isolated cleft palate is a result of which of the following?

   A. Abnormal development of first pharyngeal arch

   B. Error in development between 8 and 12 weeks of gestation

   C. Microdeletion of chromosome 22q

   D. Folic acid deficiency

   E. All of the above

HPI: A 7-year-old boy is brought to your office by his parents because of difficulty at school. They state that he is unable to concentrate in class, has delays in his speech, and is quickly falling behind his classmates. In addition, his teachers have reported aggressive and impulsive behavior, as well as difficulty interacting with his peers. The patient was born premature with a low birth weight and has had a history of poor feeding and slow growth. The mother is a recovering alcoholic who has been sober for the past 5 years but admits to drinking heavily during the pregnancy. They deny any significant family history of any diseases.

PE: The parents are both of normal build, but the child appears small for his age. His height and weight are both measured to be below the tenth percentile. HEENT exam reveals mild microcephaly, a thin upper lip, flat mid-face, and short palpebral fissures. On cardiovascular exam, a grade 2/6 holosystolic murmur is heard at the left sternal border. The remainder of his exam shows no abnormalities.

Labs: Echocardiogram shows a small VSD.

Thought Questions

- What is the most likely cause of the child's symptoms?
- How is your diagnosis made?
- What is the prognosis for the child?
- What are some other common chemical teratogens?

Basic Science Review and Discussion

Syndrome Description Fetal alcohol syndrome (FAS) describes a set of irreversible signs and symptoms found in some children as a result of the maternal ingestion of alcohol during pregnancy. Although the phenotype of FAS can be highly variable, the most common clinical features include prenatal and postnatal **growth retardation, developmental disabilities, and a distinctive facial morphology** (microcephaly, short palpebral fissures, low nasal root, and a thin upper lip). Other important findings include congenital heart defects, joint abnormalities, and structural defects in various other systems (renal, neurologic, ocular, genitourinary, hepatic, and immune systems). When the manifestations are relatively minor, the condition is known as fetal alcohol effect (FAE). There is no safe level of alcohol use in pregnancy, but the incidence of FAS increases among women with a higher alcohol intake, especially during the first trimester. As children with FAS mature, the facial features become less recognizable, but their poor social/living skills may make independent living difficult as adults.

A diagnosis is made clinically by a history of maternal alcohol use, in conjunction with the constellation of symptoms in the child. Although there is no specific treatment for FAS, it is important to evaluate the child for associated birth defects, some of which (e.g., cardiac) may be corrected surgically. Educational and community resources can be used to help support the family and help the child reach his or her fullest potential. Clinicians should recognize that this diagnosis might also be a sign of a continuing substance abuse problem in the family and the need for additional social support.

Early Embryogenesis and Organogenesis After fertilization of the ovum by the sperm, the resulting **zygote** undergoes a series of cell divisions reaching the 16-cell **morula** stage by day 4. After the morula enters the uterine cavity, the blastocyst is formed when an influx of fluid separates the morula into the inner and outer cell masses, which will give rise to the embryo and the trophoblast, respectively (Figure 41-1). The blastocyst is implanted into the endometrium by the end of the first week. By the start of week 2, the **trophoblast** begins to differentiate into the inner cytotrophoblast and the outer syncytiotrophoblast, and together they will eventually give rise to the placenta. Meanwhile, the inner cell mass divides into the **bilaminar germ disc**, composed of the epiblast and the hypoblast. During the third week of development, the embryo is primarily preoccupied with the process of **gastrulation**. This is characterized by the formation of the primitive streak on the epiblast, followed by the invagination of epiblast cells to form the three germ layers of the embryo: the inner endoderm, the middle mesoderm, and the outer ectoderm. The **endodermal layer** eventually gives rise to the GI and respiratory systems. The **mesoderm** forms the cardiovascular, musculoskeletal, and genitourinary systems. The **ectoderm layer** will differentiate into the nervous system (neural crest, neural tube), skin, and many sensory organs (hair, eyes, nose, and ears). Alcohol has been shown to be toxic to the epiblast layer and therefore can have deleterious effects on multiple organ systems, although some organs (e.g., the brain and heart) seem to be especially sensitive. The period of organogenesis primarily lasts from the third week to the eighth week of gestation and is the time when most of the major organ

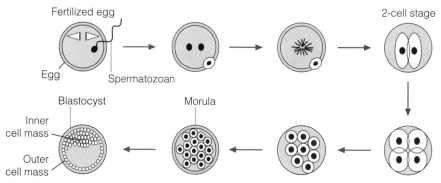

Figure 41-1 Early events in fetal development.

systems are formed. Although fetal growth retardation can occur with alcohol use during any period in pregnancy, most major defects are the result of use during the first trimester.

Classic Chemical Teratogens   Alcohol is just one of many chemicals linked to birth defects. Another classic example is **thalidomide,** which was used in the 1950s and 1960s for the treatment of nausea and insomnia. It was eventually discovered to cause major limb deformities, intestinal atresia, and cardiac defects. **Isotretinoin (Accutane)** is an analogue of

vitamin A used to treat severe acne. However, this drug also produces a characteristic set of birth defects called isotretinoin/vitamin A embryopathy. The symptoms include abnormal ear development, mandibular hypoplasia, cleft palate, and neural tube and cardiac defects. **Diethylstil-bestrol (DES)** is a synthetic estrogen that was used to prevent recurrent miscarriages in the 1940s through the 1960s. However, it was eventually found to cause early onset vaginal carcinomas and malformations of the genitourinary tract (T-shaped uterus, müllerian fusion defects) in women exposed in utero.

Case Conclusion   The diagnosis of FAS is made from the history of maternal alcohol use, characteristic facial features, and developmental abnormalities. The child was enrolled into the special education program at his elementary school, where he was able to receive greater attention and help on his language disabilities. Although he was found to have a low-normal IQ, the patient was unable to finish high school and eventually was placed in a group home for developmentally delayed adults because of his poor independent living skills.

Thumbnail: Teratogens

Chemical Teratogens	
Teratogen	**Symptoms**
Alcohol	Craniofacial abnormalities, growth retardation, developmental delay, cardiovascular abnormalities (VSDs)
Thalidomide	Limb agenesis/deformities, intestinal atresia, cardiac abnormalities
Isotretinoin	Ear abnormalities, cleft palate, mandibular hypoplasia, neural tube and cardiac defects
DES	Genitourinary cancers and malformations

Key Points

- The stages of early embryo development include fertilization → cleavage and formation of morula → blastocyst → implantation → formation of bilaminar disc (epiblast and hypoblast) → gastrulation and formation of trilaminar germ disc.

- Inner cell mass:
  epiblast → ectoderm, mesoderm, endoderm
  hypoblast → yolk sac

- Outer cell mass → trophoblast → cytotrophoblast, syncytiotrophoblast → placenta

- Ectoderm forms the nervous system, ear, nose, eyes, and skin.

- Mesoderm forms the musculoskeletal, cardiovascular, and genitourinary systems.

- Endoderm forms the gastrointestinal and respiratory tracts.

Questions

1. A 1-year-old girl is diagnosed with FAS and found to have the characteristic facial features and the coordination difficulties, hearing loss, and a diffusely cloudy cornea. Which germinal layer(s) seem to be affected?

   A. Mesoderm
   B. Endoderm
   C. Ectoderm
   D. Endoderm and ectoderm
   E. Endoderm and mesoderm

2. Most birth defects arise during the period of organogenesis between the third and eighth weeks of development. However, within that time span, each organ system is susceptible to environmental insults at specific times. For example, limb formation reaches a critical state around the fifth week of gestation when the limb buds appear. Which of the following teratogens would you be most worried about because of its effects on bone development?

   A. Isotretinoin
   B. Thalidomide
   C. Lithium
   D. Alcohol
   E. DES

3. Organogenesis cannot begin without the proper formation of the three germ layers (i.e., the ectoderm, mesoderm, and endoderm). Which of the following terms describes the events in the third week of development that establish these three layers?

   A. Cleavage
   B. Invagination
   C. Migration
   D. Compaction
   E. Gastrulation

HPI: AC comes to your office for a second opinion after learning the results of her obstetric US. She is a healthy 28-year-old female currently at 19 weeks of gestation. This is her first pregnancy, which was unplanned but desired. Her maternal serum prenatal screening at 16 weeks was abnormal, with an elevated maternal serum AFP (MSAFP) of 3.4 multiples of the median (MoM), which prompted further testing. Last week, she had a detailed US examination revealing a live single fetus appropriately grown for gestational age with a Chiari II malformation (Lemon and/or Banana sign, Figure 42-1) and lumbosacral myelomeningocele (Figure 42-2).
She reports no past significant illnesses. AC has being taking prenatal vitamins since her first visit at 12 weeks. She denies any tobacco, alcohol, or illicit drug use, past or current.

Thought Questions

- What are the objectives of second-trimester prenatal screening? When are they done?

- What is the critical time period for neural tube closure?

- What are the known predisposing factors for neural tube defects (NTDs)?

Basic Science Review and Discussion

Maternal Serum Screening   **Maternal serum screening** in the second trimester of pregnancy is routinely offered to all pregnant women in the United States. It is a screening test for **Down syndrome** and **NTDs,** identifying a population at risk (screen positive) and a low-risk population. Additionally, a variety of other problems can also be identified, such as other chromosomal abnormalities and abdominal wall defects, but at lower detection rates (sensitivity). Using three analytes (AFP, unconjugated estriol, and hCG), it can detect 60% of Down syndrome cases (decreased AFP, decreased estriol, and increased hCG) and more than 90% of open NTDs (increased AFP) among low-risk women, using a fixed cutoff of 5% (false positive). The test is done between 15 and 20 weeks of gestation and is most effective between **16 and 18 weeks.** Those women who are screen positive need to undergo further testing.

Neural Tube Development   The **formation of the neural tube** begins between days 22 and 23 of gestation (fourth week) in the region of the fourth and sixth somites. Fusion of the neural folds occurs in cranial and caudal directions, probably at **multisite initiation.** The anterior neuropore (future brain) closes by day 25 and the posterior pore (future spinal cord) closes by day 27. Closure of the neural tube coincides with establishment of its vascular supply. Most NTDs develop as a result of defective closure at the fourth week of development (sixth week of gestation or from the LMP) (Figure 42-3).

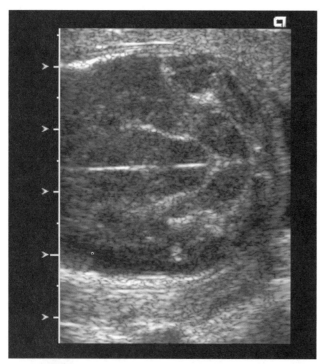

Figure 42-1 Banana sign. Note the cerebellum pulled posteriorly into a banana shape. (Courtesy Dr. Peter Callen, Department of Radiology, and Obstetrics, Gynecology and Reproductive Sciences, UCSF.)

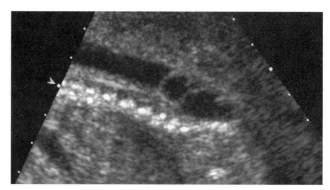

Figure 42-2 Lumbosacral myelomeningocele. Note the bubble of epithelium poking through the neural tube defect and the skin disruption at the saral level. (Courtesy Dr. Peter Callen, Department of Radiology, and Obstetrics, Gynecology and Reproductive Sciences, UCSF.)

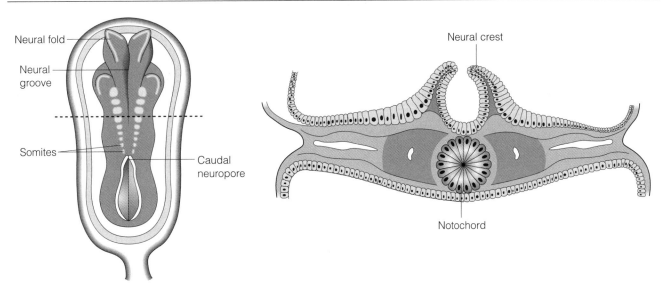

Figure 42-3 Neural tube development.

Etiology of NTDs   NTDs are a classic example of **multifactorial inheritance (MFI),** emphasizing the interactions between environmental and genetic factors. Geographic and ethnic variations may reflect environmental and genetic factors to the occurrence of **NTDs.** Variations in the incidence of NTDs related to seasonal or temporal changes in the same region and among different areas in homogeneous populations support environmental contribution. Decreased levels of folic acid have been found among mothers who gave birth to babies with NTDs. Supplementation with periconceptional folic acid effectively reduces the incidence of recurrence of NTDs, as well as first occurrence, as shown by randomized controlled trials (RCTs). Doubling of the risk of NTDs has been associated with homozygosity for a common mutation in the gene for MTHFR, the C677T allelic variant, which encodes an enzyme with reduced activity. However, even if the association were causal, this MTHFR variant would account for only a small fraction of NTDs prevented by folic acid. The risk of NTDs seen with certain genotypes may vary depending on maternal factors, such as the blood levels of vitamin B_{12} or folate.

Case Conclusion   AC and her partner decide to terminate this pregnancy after genetic counseling. Chromosome studies of the fetus reveal a normal 46,XY karyotype. An autopsy confirmed the presence of a large lumbosacral myelomeningocele. No additional major or minor anomalies were noted.

Thumbnail: Neural Development

Spinal Cord and Brain Development

In embryology, the age of the embryo/fetus is given from the time of conception, whereas in clinical practice gestational age is derived from the LMP.

The neural tube gives rise to the CNS, consisting of brain and spinal cord.

The neural crest gives rise to the peripheral nervous system (PNS) and autonomic nervous system (ANS).

Formation of the neural tube (neurulation) begins 22 to 23 days in the region of the fourth and sixth pairs of somites.

The cranial two thirds of the neural plate and tube down to the fourth pair of somites represents the brain, and the caudal one third of the neural plate and tube (below the fourth pair of somites) represents the future spinal cord.

The neural tube likely closes in a multisite fashion. Closure of the neural tube proceeds in the cranial and caudal direction until small areas at the ends remain open, the rostral and the caudal neurospores. By day 25 of development, the rostral neurospore closes, and by day 27, the caudal neurospore does.

Key Points

- NTDs are one of the most common major malformations. Isolated NTDs, as well as other isolated single organ malformations, are explained by MFI.

- Families with prior affected offspring with NTDs are at an increased risk of recurrence (10-fold over baseline). Periconceptional use of folic acid can reduce the incidence and the recurrence of NTDs.

- Drugs (valproic acid), hyperthermia, single-gene defects, and chromosomal abnormalities have been associated with NTDs. The recurrence risks in these cases are different from those for MFI and must be individualized.

Questions

1. For this couple's next pregnancy, the greatest risk reduction of recurrence of NTDs is achieved by which of the following?
   A. FDA daily recommended allowance of folic acid (0.4 mg)
   B. High dose of folic acid periconceptionally (4 mg)
   C. Adoption, the risk of recurrence is too great
   D. Avoid alcohol consumption
   E. Avoid exposure to x-rays

2. Most NTDs are the result of which of the following?
   A. Teratogen exposure
   B. Vitamin deficiency
   C. Multifactorial etiology
   D. Single-gene defects
   E. Chromosomal abnormalities

3. A 20-year-old woman with seizure disorder on valproic acid has a positive pregnancy test 1 day after she missed her period. Regarding the teratogenic risk of the medication, how would you counsel her?
   A. The risk of NTDs is probably only slightly increased over background risk (1/1500) if she stops taking valproic acid now.
   B. The risk of NTDs secondary to valproic acid intake is not increased.
   C. Risk of NTDs is 10- to 20-fold over background (6%) with exposure during the first trimester.
   D. Continue taking valproic acid, because the damage has already been done.
   E. A and C are correct

HPI: A 15-year-old boy is referred to the cardiologist for hypertension found during a routine physical exam. The patient notes no symptoms from the high BP but does complain of a long history of weakness and pain in both legs after mild exercise. He has been quite healthy and denies any significant family history of illness.

PE: BP 145/95 mm Hg (arms) and 80/40 mm Hg (legs), HR 85 beats/min, RR 12 breaths/min

The child appears well developed and in no acute distress. On cardiovascular exam, a grade 3/6 systolic ejection murmur is heard at the suprasternal notch. Systolic murmurs can also be heard over the left and right sides of the chest, both laterally and posteriorly. Extremity exam reveals bounding carotid and radial pulses, and the lower extremity (femoral, popliteal, posterior tibial, and dorsalis pedis) pulses are weak. The remainder of the exam shows no abnormalities.

Labs: Chest x-ray shows a moderately enlarged heart with notching of the ribs. ECG reveals a left-axis deviation, suggestive of left ventricular hypertrophy. Echocardiogram demonstrates a bicuspid aortic valve and decreased flow through the descending aorta.

Thought Questions

- What is the diagnosis?
- What is the developmental process that forms the major arterial system?
- Which part of the embryologic system gives rise to this defect?
- How is this condition treated?

Basic Science Review and Discussion

Syndrome Description **Coarctation of the aorta** is a congenital malformation that involves the abnormal **thickening of the aortic wall** that can cause the narrowing of the lumen anywhere from the transverse arch to the origin of the iliac arteries (Figure 43-1). An overwhelming majority (98%) occurs just distal to the ductus arteriosus. Coarctation can

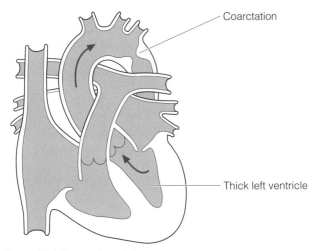

Figure 43-1 Coarctation of the aorta.

develop alone or in conjunction with other cardiac abnormalities including bicuspid aortic valve, VSD, or transverse arch hypoplasia. The classic symptoms of coarctation are **unequal BPs and pulses** between the upper and lower extremities. Some children may also experience pain or weakness in the lower extremities with exercise. A systolic ejection murmur may indicate the presence of a bicuspid aortic valve, and flow murmurs along the lateral thoracic region are consistent with increased collateral circulation. Infants who are symptomatic generally have severe coarctation and can present with symptoms of heart failure, acidosis, and insufficient perfusion of the lower extremities.

Chest X-ray may show an enlarged cardiac silhouette due to ventricular hypertrophy, as well as rib notching from pressure erosion by enlarged collateral vessels. Left-axis deviation and ventricular hypertrophy can also be seen on ECG. The diagnosis can be confirmed by an echocardiogram, which can visualize the segment of narrowed blood flow and detect other cardiac abnormalities. Treatment is by surgical correction of the defect either through excision of the area of coarctation or enlargement with a prosthetic patch. If untreated, most patients will experience chronic systemic hypertension with associated complications of intracranial hemorrhage, coronary artery disease, and heart failure. In neonates with severe disease, heart failure and lower extremity cyanosis may be fatal if not treated immediately.

Pharyngeal (Branchial) Arches The pharyngeal arches appear around the fourth to fifth weeks and are crucial in the development of the head and neck region (Figure 43-2). The arches are composed of **mesenchymal** and **neural crest cells** that are sandwiched between surface ectoderm (**pharyngeal cleft**) and a layer of endodermal epithelium (**pharyngeal pouches**). Each pharyngeal arch has its own artery (called **aortic arches**) and cranial nerve, which gives rise to distinctive skeletal and muscular components of the head and neck. The **first pharyngeal arch** gives rise to the mandible and maxilla and contributes to the formation of the bones of the middle ear (e.g., incus and malleus). The muscles of mastication (e.g., temporal, masseter, and pterygoids) are also derived from the first arch and are innervated by the mandibular branch of the trigeminal nerve. The **second pharyngeal arch** produces the stapes and lesser horn of the hyoid bone, as well as the muscles of facial expression, the stapedius, stylohyoid, and posterior belly of the digastric. The nervous innervation of these muscles is through the facial nerve. The **third pharyngeal arch** forms the greater horn of the hyoid bone. The musculature of this arch is the stylopharyngeus muscle that is innervated by the glossopharyngeal nerve. The **fourth and sixth arches** eventually fuse to give rise to the thyroid, cricoid, arytenoid, corniculate, and cuneiform cartilages. The fourth arch also develops into the cricothyroid, levator veli palatini, and pharyngeal constrictor muscles, and the sixth arch forms all of the intrinsic muscles of the larynx (except the cricothyroid). The muscles of the fourth arch are supplied by the superior laryngeal branch of the vagus, and the muscles of the sixth arch are innervated by the recurrent laryngeal branch.

Pharyngeal (Branchial) Cleft Pharyngeal clefts are composed of **ectoderm tissue.** Of those present at 5 weeks of gestation, only one makes a major developmental contribution. The **first cleft** gives rise to the external auditory meatus, and the other clefts form a temporary cervical sinus that disappears with the growth of the second arch.

Pharyngeal (Branchial) Pouches The five pairs of pharyngeal pouches are composed of **endodermal** epithelium that develops into several important organs. The **first pouch** is involved in the creation of the middle ear, eustachian tube, and the tympanic membrane. The **second pouch** forms the epithelial lining of the palatine tonsil. The dorsal wing of the **third pouch** develops into the inferior parathyroid gland, and the ventral wing differentiates into the thymus. The thymus eventually migrates medially and caudally while pulling the inferior parathyroid gland to its dorsal surface. The **fourth pouch** differentiates into the superior parathy-

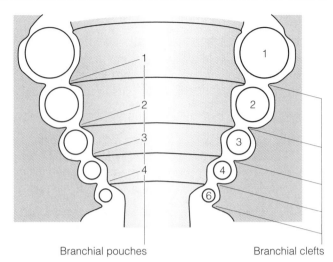

Figure 43-2 Coronal section of the embryonic pharynx (arches are the circles numbered 1 through 6).

Branchial pouches   Branchial clefts

roid gland, and the **fifth pouch** (usually considered part of the fourth pouch) gives rise to the ultimobranchial body of the thyroid. These cells develop into the parafollicular or C-cells that secrete calcitonin.

Aortic Arches The aortic arches are derived from the aortic sac at the distal end of the truncus arteriosus and during development, each is paired with a pharyngeal arch. The **first aortic arch** has mostly regressed by the end of the fourth week, with only a small portion remaining to form the maxillary artery. The **second arch** develops into the hyoid and stapedial arteries. The **third aortic arch** gives rise to the common carotid artery, the external carotid artery, and the beginning of the internal carotid artery. On the left side, the **fourth arch** forms the aortic arch, whereas on the right side, it differentiates into the proximal right subclavian artery. The **sixth aortic arch** is also known as the **pulmonary arch,** because the right side develops into the proximal right pulmonary artery and left side forms the ductus arteriosus. Coarctation of the aorta is caused by the abnormal development of the fourth aortic arch, which leads to thickening of the aortic wall and narrowing of the lumen.

Case Conclusion The patient was found to have a bicuspid aortic valve and mild stenosis of the aorta just distal to the origin of the left subclavian artery. The area of the coarctation was excised and repaired by an end-to-end anastomosis of the transverse aorta and the descending aorta. After the operation, the patient was found to have markedly increased lower extremity pulsations and increased perfusion.

Thumbnail: Branchial Arch Anomalies

Head, Neck, and Arterial Development

Pharyngeal arch derivatives:

Pharyngeal arch	Nerve	Skeleton	Muscles
First (mandibular)	CN V$_3$	Mandible, maxilla, middle ear (incus, malleus)	Mastication (temporal, masseter, medial/lateral pterygoids)
Second (hyoid)	CN VII	Stapes, hyoid (lesser horn)	Facial expression, stapedius, stylohyoid
Third	CN IX	Hyoid (greater horn)	Stylopharyngeus
Fourth and sixth	CN X	Thyroid, cricoid, arytenoids, corniculate, cuneiform cartilages	Cricothyroid, levator veli palatini, constrictors (fourth); intrinsic muscles of larynx (sixth)

Pharyngeal pouch derivatives:

Pharyngeal pouch	Derivative
First	Middle ear, eustachian tube, tympanic membrane
Second	Epithelial lining of palatine
Third	Thymus (ventral wing), inferior parathyroid gland (dorsal wing)
Fourth	Superior parathyroid gland
Fifth	Ultimobranchial body (parafollicular cells of the thyroid)

Aortic arch derivatives:

Aortic arch	Derivative
First	Maxillary artery
Second	Hyoid artery, stapedial artery
Third	Common carotid artery, proximal internal carotid artery, external carotid artery
Fourth	Aortic arch (left), proximal right subclavian artery (right)
Sixth	Ductus arteriosus (left), proximal right pulmonary artery (right)

Key Points

▶ The first pharyngeal cleft gives rise to the external auditory meatus.

▶ The fifth pharyngeal and aortic arches do not make significant contributions to embryologic development.

Questions

1. DiGeorge's syndrome is a constellation of congenital defects that includes hypoplasia of the thymus and the inferior and superior parathyroid glands. Based on these symptoms, which of the following embryologic structures are involved?

   A. Second and third pharyngeal arches
   B. Third and fourth pharyngeal pouches
   C. First pharyngeal cleft
   D. Second and third aortic arches
   E. Fourth and fifth pharyngeal pouches

2. A neonate is diagnosed with hemifacial microsomia. This disorder comprises a number of craniofacial malformations including small and flattened maxillary, temporal, and zygomatic bones. What type of tissue is involved in this abnormality?

   A. Ectoderm
   B. Endoderm
   C. Mesoderm
   D. Ectoderm and mesoderm
   E. Neural crest

3. The vocal cords are controlled by the intrinsic muscles of the larynx. Two patients are separately seen in your clinic for symptoms of hoarseness. Both patients have neck masses, but the lesions impinge on different nerves and affect different muscles. Which of the following statements is true about the embryology involved in these cases?

   A. The derivatives of the second and fourth pharyngeal arches are involved.
   B. One patient has dysfunction of the cricothyroid muscle, which is derived from the sixth arch and supplied by the recurrent laryngeal nerve.
   C. The levator palatini is the only intrinsic muscle of the larynx not supplied by the recurrent laryngeal nerve.
   D. Both masses affect the intrinsic muscles of the larynx, which are all derived from the sixth arch.
   E. One of the lesions affects the cricothyroid muscle that is innervated by the superior laryngeal nerve and derived from the fourth pharyngeal arch.

HPI: A 10-month-old girl presents to your office with failure to thrive. The parents state that the pregnancy was uncomplicated and she was delivered at term with average weight and height for her gestational age. A faint murmur was detected in the nursery, but the baby otherwise seemed to be healthy and was sent home. Over the past few months though, she has had increasingly poor appetite and frequently becomes short of breath and tired after only a short time at play. The child's growth seems to have slowed and she is falling behind developmentally, compared with other children her age. Her parents deny any significant family history of illness.

PE: BP 90/65, HR 135 beats/min, RR 30 breaths/min

The child appears small for her age and has a faintly pale skin color at rest that deepens with crying. Her height and weight are both measured to be around the twenty-fifth percentile. HEENT exam reveals blue-tinged lips. On cardiovascular exam, a heave can be felt midline below the xiphoid process and a grade 3/6 systolic ejection murmur is heard at the left upper sternal border. The remainder of her exam shows no abnormalities.

Labs: Chest x-ray shows a right-sided aortic arch and an elevated, rounded apex that causes the heart silhouette to resemble the shape of a boot. ECG reveals a right-axis deviation, suggestive of right ventricular hypertrophy. Echocardiogram shows an interventricular septal defect and decreased blood flow through the pulmonary artery.

Thought Questions

- What is the diagnosis?
- What is the developmental error that causes this defect?
- How is this condition treated?
- What is the prognosis for this patient without treatment?

Basic Science Review and Discussion

Syndrome Description Tetralogy of Fallot is caused by the abnormal development of the conotruncal septum, which results in the four characteristic signs: (1) **pulmonary stenosis,** (2) **overriding aorta,** (3) **interventricular septal defect,** and (4) **hypertrophy of the right ventricle** resulting from the increased pressure on the right side of the heart (Figure 44-1). The etiology of this syndrome is multifactorial and includes both genetic mutations (chromosome 22q11 deletion) and environmental insults (e.g., drugs and alcohol). Symptoms depend on the degree of right ventricular outflow obstruction. When severe pulmonary stenosis is present, cyanosis can be detected immediately after birth. In children with less severe disease, cyanosis may appear later in life and be most easily seen in the mucous membranes of the lips and fingernails. Children will also complain of dyspnea on exertion and will need to rest after only a short period of activity. Patients with untreated disease may experience retardations of growth and development including a delay in the onset of puberty. On exam, the child will usually have normal BPs and pulse, but a harsh systolic murmur is usually heard along the left sternal

border. Other exam findings may include a right ventricular impulse and a systolic thrill along the left sternal border.

On x-ray, the heart will be of normal size, but a right-sided aortic arch will be present, as well as an elevated apical shadow from the hypertrophied right ventricle, causing the comparison of the heart silhouette to a boot. An ECG can detect a right-axis deviation due to the increased electrical activity of the enlarged right ventricle. An echocardiogram confirms the diagnosis and can reveal the severity of the VSD and the pulmonary artery stenosis. Definitive treatment is through corrective surgery to close the VSD and the

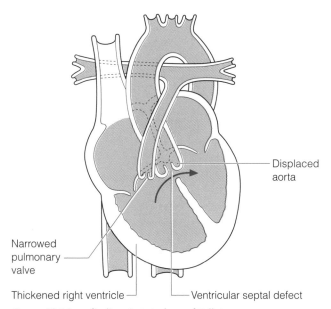

Figure 44-1 Four findings in tetralogy of Fallot.

Displaced aorta

Narrowed pulmonary valve

Thickened right ventricle

Ventricular septal defect

removal of muscle to relieve the pulmonary stenosis. When a neonate presents with severe right ventricular outflow tract obstruction, treatment may include a systemic-to-pulmonary artery shunt to increase blood flow to the lungs before attempting corrective surgery later in infancy. Before treatment became available, children with tetralogy of Fallot usually had increasing cyanosis and exercise intolerance with shortened life spans. After successful surgery, patients are generally able to lead normal lives.

Cardiac Development: Formation of the Heart Tube   The cardiovascular system is derived from the **mesoderm layer** of the trilaminar germ layer formed after gastrulation. Development begins during the **third week of gestation** when an angiogenic cell cluster forms at the anterior central portion of the embryo. As the embryo folds cephalocaudally, the cardiogenic area also folds into a **heart tube.** Even at this early stage, the embryonic heart tube is already receiving venous flow from its caudal end and pumping blood through the first aortic arch and into the dorsal aorta. At the same time, mesoderm around the endocardial tube form the three layers of the heart wall, composed of an **outer epicardium,** a muscular wall of **myocardium,** and the **endocardium** that is the internal endothelial lining. Between days 23 and 28, the heart tube elongates and bends to create the cardiac loop with a common atrium and a narrow atrioventricular junction connecting it to the primitive ventricle. The **bulbus cordis** is the caudal section of the heart tube and will eventually form three structures: The proximal third will form the trabeculated part of the right ventricle, the midportion (conus cordis) will form the outflow tracts of the ventricles, and the distal segment (truncus arteriosus) will eventually give rise to the proximal portions of the aorta and the pulmonary artery (Figure 44-2).

Cardiac Development: Formation of the Septa   Between days 27 and 37, the heart continues to develop through the formation of the major septa. Septum formation is achieved through the formation of tissue, called endocardial cushions, which subdivide the lumen into two cavities. The right and left atria are created by the formation of the **septum primum** and **septum secundum** that subdivides the primitive atrium while allowing for an interatrial opening (foramen ovale) to continue the right-to-left shunting of blood. At the end of the fourth week, endocardial cushions also appear in the atrioventricular canal to form the right and left canals, as well as the mitral and tricuspid valves. During this time, the medial walls of the ventricles gradually fuse to form the muscular interventricular septum. The conus cordis comprises the middle third of the bulbus cordis, and during the fifth week of development, cushions subdivide the conus to form the outflow tract of the right and left ventricles, as well as the membranous portion of the interventricular septum. Cushions also appear in the truncus arteriosus (distal third of bulbus cordis) and grow in a spiral pattern to form the aorticopulmonary septum and divide the truncus into the aortic and pulmonary tracts.

Congenital Heart Disease   Congenital heart disease (CHD) is an abnormality of cardiac structure and function that is present at birth. VSD is the most common CHD, followed by atrial septal defect (ASD), and patent ductus arteriosus (PDA). Other cardiac malformations include transposition of the great vessels, truncus arteriosus, and coarctation of the aorta. Although most congenital heart defects are isolated occurrences, some may be a manifestation of a more complex disease (e.g., Down, Turner's, or Marfan's syndromes) or a teratogen (e.g., alcohol, rubella, or retinoic acid).

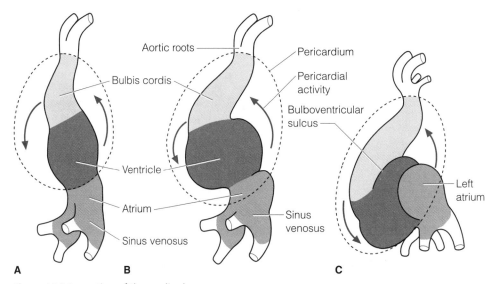

Figure 44-2 Formation of the cardiac loop.

Case Conclusion   The infant first underwent a successful palliative procedure to place an aortopulmonary shunt that resolved her immediate symptoms. At 2 years of age, she is doing well and is scheduled for corrective repair, which involves resection of the pulmonic stenosis and patch closure of the interventricular septal defect.

Thumbnail: Cardiac Development

Time Line of Cardiac Development

Time period	Development
Third week	Angiogenic cell cluster appears; heart tube forms; three layers of the heart wall are created
Day 23 to 28	Heart tube transforms into the cardiac loop
Day 27 to 37	Formation of the cardiac septa
Postnatal	Closure of the foramen ovale

Key Points

▶ Tetralogy of Fallot is composed of the following four findings:
1. Pulmonary stenosis
2. Overriding aorta
3. Interventricular septal defect
4. Hypertrophy of the right ventricle

▶ The bulbus cordis forms the following structures:
1. Proximal portion: trabeculated part of right ventricle
2. Middle portion (conus cordis): ventricular outflow tracts
3. Distal portion (truncus arteriosus): trunk and proximal part of the aorta and pulmonary artery

Questions

1. Tetralogy of Fallot is one of many congenital diseases caused by the abnormal development of the bulbus cordis. Which of the following conditions arises from the failure of the conotruncal septum to form and descend?

   A. Transposition of the great vessels
   B. Persistent truncus arteriosus
   C. Aortic and pulmonary valvular stenosis
   D. Tetralogy of Fallot
   E. Dextrocardia

2. An infant with tetralogy of Fallot and severe right ventricular outflow obstruction is transferred to the cardiac care unit of your hospital for surgery to correct the defects. While waiting for the procedure, she becomes progressively hypoxic due to the closure of the PDA supplying blood to her pulmonary vasculature. Which of the following drugs would you administer to prevent the closure of the ductus arteriosus while waiting for the surgery?

   A. Ibuprofen
   B. Dexamethasone
   C. PGE_1 (Prostaglandin E_1)
   D. TXA_2 (Thromboxane)
   E. Indomethacin

3. While examining a fetus in distress, you find that the developing heart has gross hypertrophy of the right atrium and ventricle, as well as an underdeveloped left side of the heart. You speculate that this is due to the decreased blood flow into the left atrium caused by which of the following?

   A. Absence of the atrial septum
   B. Premature fusion of the septum primum and septum secundum
   C. Inadequate development of the septum secundum
   D. Failure of the endocardial cushions to fuse
   E. Patent foramen ovale

HPI: The pediatrics team is called emergently to the delivery suite for a newborn in respiratory distress. The baby was a product of a normal vaginal delivery. The mother states that she has three other children but never sought out prenatal care because the course of the pregnancy appeared to be normal. The other children are healthy and the parents deny any significant family history of illness.

PE: HR 125 beats/min, RR 50 breaths/min, O_2 Sat 87%

The baby is markedly tachypneic and only crying faintly. HEENT exam reveals nasal flaring and blue-tinged lips. On chest exam, there is moderate intercostal retractions and use of accessory muscles of respiration. Clear breath sounds can be heard over the right lung field and soft bowel sounds can be heard over the left lung field. No murmurs are present and the remainder of her exam shows no abnormalities. Chest x-ray shows a normal-appearing lung in the right side of the chest and air-filled bowel in the left with displacement of the mediastinum to the right.

Thought Questions

- What is the diagnosis?
- What are the steps involved in the formation of the diaphragm and lungs?
- What developmental error causes this defect?
- How is this condition treated?

Basic Science Review and Discussion

Syndrome Description   **Congenital diaphragmatic hernia (CDH)** occurs as a result of a defect in the pleuroperitoneal fold, allowing bowel to enter the thoracic cavity. This herniation occurs predominantly on the left side (85%) and prevents normal lung development, especially in the ipsilateral lung. Shortly after birth, the neonate will experience respiratory distress. This is caused by distension of the bowel with swallowed air that compresses both the contralateral lung and the hypoplastic ipsilateral lung. Associated symptoms include tachypnea, cyanosis, use of accessory muscles of respiration, and the presence of bowel sounds in the chest. About half of infants with CDH also have other congenital malformations, especially involving the cardiac and genitourinary systems.

A diagnosis can be made as early as 15 weeks of gestation by ultrasound. An x-ray demonstrating air-filled bowel above the diaphragm is confirmatory. Treatment includes ventilatory support of the neonate and surgical repair of the defect with reduction of the herniated bowel. The survival rate in these infants is approximately 35% to 50% and is dependent on the degree of lung hypoplasia and the severity of associated malformations (Figures 45-1 and 45-2).

Development of the Diaphragm   The diaphragm is composed of four components: **septum transversum, pleuroperitoneal folds, body wall,** and **esophagus mesentery** (Figures 45-3).

By the end of the third week of gestation, the tendinous septum transversum is present to incompletely separate the thoracic and abdominal cavities. As the lung buds grow and develop, the caudal border of the pleural cavity (pleuroperitoneal folds) extends and fuses with the septum transversum and the esophageal mesentery. The pleural cavity continues to expand, and after contact with the body wall, a rim of myoblasts infiltrates the membrane to form the muscular segment of the diaphragm.

Pulmonary Embryology   The **lung bud** (respiratory diverticulum) first appears around 4 weeks of gestation and is derived from the ventral wall of the foregut. Shortly thereafter, the **esophagotracheal ridges** appear and fuse to divide the foregut into the esophagus as the dorsal segment and the trachea and lung buds as the ventral portion. At the beginning of the fifth week, the right and left main bronchial buds begin to grow from the lung bud. As the bronchial buds continue to branch, the visceral and

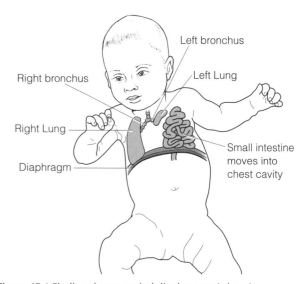

Figure 45-1 Findings in congenital diaphragmatic hernia.

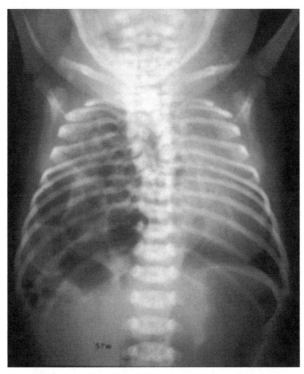

Figure 45-2 X-ray showing air-filled bowel in the right chest. (Copyright-protected material used with permission of the author and the University of Iowa's Virtual Hospital, www.vh.org.)

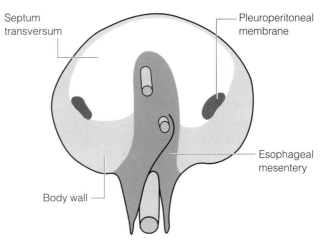

Figure 45-3 Components of the diaphragm.

parietal pleura develop from the mesodermal layers covering the outside of the lung and the body wall, respectively. By the sixth month, the respiratory bronchioles and alveolar ducts have formed and will undergo further development into terminal sacs. This occurs when the cuboidal epithelium transitions into thin squamous epithelium **(type I alveolar epithelial cells)** that becomes closely associated with blood and lymph capillaries. In the last few months before birth, **type II alveolar cells** appear and begin secreting surfactant. The lungs continue to develop even after birth as the alveoli mature and increase severalfold in number.

Case Conclusion   The infant was transferred to the pediatric ICU where she responded well to ventilatory support. The patient underwent surgery to correct a 4-cm diaphragmatic defect and to reduce the transverse colon that was herniating into the chest. Her condition improved dramatically after the operation, and she is feeding and recovering well.

Thumbnail: Pulmonary Development

Time Line of Pulmonary Development	
Time period	**Development**
Week 4	Lung bud appears from foregut
Week 5	Right and left bronchial buds grow from lung bud
Weeks 5 to 16	Continued branching to create terminal bronchioles
Weeks 16 to 26	Respiratory bronchioles and alveolar ducts appear
Weeks 26 to birth	Primitive alveoli form
Neonate to childhood	Formation and maturation of alveoli

Key Points

▶ The diaphragm is derived from the following four structures:

1. Septum transversum

2. Two pleuroperitoneal membranes

3. Muscular ingrowth from the body wall

4. Esophagus mesentery

Questions

1. Premature infants are at high risk for respiratory distress syndrome (RDS), a disease that contributes to approximately one fifth of all neonatal mortality. The immature lungs are unable to overcome the air-fluid surface tension, causing collapse of the alveoli during expiration. What is the main cause of this syndrome?

   A. Insufficient numbers of alveoli
   B. Inadequate function of type II alveolar cells
   C. Inadequate function of type I alveolar cells
   D. Inadequate respiratory musculature
   E. Increased hyaline membrane formation

2. The epithelium of the larynx, trachea, and bronchi are all derived from the original lung bud that grows from the primitive foregut. Which other structure originates from the same germ layer (ectoderm, endoderm, mesoderm) as the lung epithelium?

   A. Pancreas
   B. Heart
   C. Lens of the eye
   D. Kidney
   E. Spleen

3. Although the laryngeal epithelium is derived from the endodermal germ layer, the muscles of the larynx are created from mesodermal cells and are innervated by branches of the vagus nerve (CN X). What is the embryologic origin of this musculature?

   A. Fourth and sixth pharyngeal pouches
   B. First pharyngeal cleft
   C. Fourth and sixth pharyngeal arches
   D. Third pharyngeal pouch
   E. Third pharyngeal arch

HPI: On routine obstetric US at 20 weeks of gestation a large anterior abdominal wall defect is identified. Much of the liver is protruding into the abdomen. A complete anatomic survey of the fetus reveals no other identifiable anomaly. You discuss with your patient the sonographic findings and counsel her that an amniocentesis is recommended to rule out chromosomal abnormalities in the fetus. The fetal karyotype showed a normal 46,XX complement. Your patient decided to continue the pregnancy, and a recommendation was made for delivery at a tertiary care center. She delivered at term after an uncomplicated vaginal delivery. A three-generation family pedigree was reviewed and was noncontributory.

PE: Full-term, male infant in no acute distress with a large, midline abdominal wall defect with herniation of bowel and liver. A thin membrane covers the herniated contents. A systematic examination of the infant did not reveal any other major or minor anomalies.

Tests: Sonogram of the fetus, cross section of the abdomen, shows an anterior abdominal wall defect with liver and bowel protruding through the abdomen. A thin membrane is seen covering the herniated contents.

Thought Questions

- What is the diagnosis?
- What are the steps involved in the return of the midgut to the abdomen?
- What is the developmental error that causes this defect?
- How is this condition treated?

Basic Science Review and Discussion

Syndrome Description An **omphalocele** is a defect of the anterior abdominal wall that occurs in approximately 1 in 5000 births. A thin membrane, which is composed of peritoneum and amnion, covers this defect and the **umbilical cord inserts into the sac.** Omphaloceles typically contain bowel and/or liver. **Associated anomalies are common,** occurring in as many as 50% to 70% of cases. Chromosomal abnormalities (especially trisomies) are common when an omphalocele contains only bowel. Many genetic syndromes can be associated with omphalocele, but the most characteristic is **Beckwith-Wiedemann syndrome,** which is characterized by overgrowth, omphalocele, macroglossia, and ear pits. **The prognosis in omphaloceles largely depends on the presence or absence of concomitant abnormalities and the karyotype.** Isolated omphaloceles have a favorable prognosis.

Surgical repair is needed soon after birth. Attempt is made to close the defect at the time of surgery, but sometimes this is not possible. If the omphalocele is large, a silo is placed. A **silo** is a covering placed over the abdominal organs on the outside of the baby. Gradually, the organs are squeezed through the silo into the opening and returned to the abdominal cavity. Extremely large omphaloceles are not surgically repaired until the baby grows.

The main differential diagnosis is **gastroschisis,** a relatively small, right-sided paraumbilical defect through which eviscerated bowel floats within the amniotic fluid. There is no sac. Unlike omphalocele, gastroschisis is usually an isolated defect (Figures 46-1 and 46-2).

Development of the Midgut The small intestine (including most of the duodenum), the cecum, appendix, ascending colon, and two thirds of the transverse are all irrigated by the superior mesenteric artery. At the **beginning of the sixth week, the midgut protrudes into the proximal aspect of the umbilical cord (physiologic umbilical herniation)** due to the rapid growth of the midgut and relative lack of space due to a large liver and kidneys. While in the umbilical cord, the **midgut undergoes a 90-degree rotation around the axis of the superior mesenteric artery.** During the **tenth week, the intestines return to the abdomen.** Failure of the

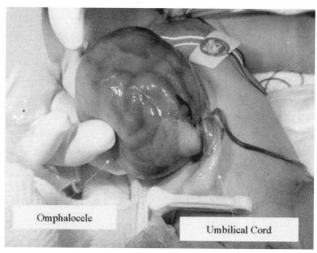

Figure 46-1 Newborn with omphalocele. (Courtesy The Fetal Treatment Center, UCSF.)

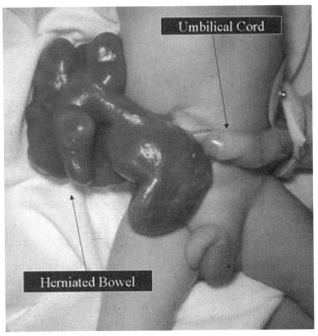

Figure 46-2 Newborn with gastroschisis. (Courtesy The Fetal Treatment Center, UCSF.)

intestines to return results in an omphalocele. Gastroschisis results from the incomplete migration of the lateral folds during the fourth week of development. Exposures that result in a decrease in vascular supply may be involved in the pathogenesis of gastroschisis.

Digestive System Embryology The primordial gut forms during the fourth week from part of the yolk sac that is incorporated into the embryo as it folds. The **endoderm of the primordial gut** gives rise to most of the epithelium of the digestive tract and the parenchyma of the glands including liver and pancreas, with the exception of the **cranial and caudal ends of the tract which are of ectodermal origin,** and the **spleen that is derived from mesenchymal cells.** The muscle layer and the connective tissue are derived from the splanchnic mesenchyme. The primordial gut is divided into the foregut, midgut, and hindgut.

Case Conclusion   The infant underwent primary surgical closure of the defect on his first day of life. His postoperative course was uncomplicated, and he was able to feed and was discharged on day 5. Two years later, he is still developing well.

Thumbnail: Gastrointestinal Embryology

Time Line of Digestive Development

Time period	Development
Week 4	Primitive gut is closed by the oropharyngeal membrane and cloacal membrane
Weeks 6 through 10	Liver hematopoiesis begins at 6 weeks; the liver is big during this time
Week 7	Cloaca is divided by the urorectal septum; the anal membrane ruptures by the eighth week
Week 10	Intestines return to abdominal cavity
Week 12	Endocrine function of pancreas begins

Key Points

▶ The digestive tract is derived from the following germ layers:

1. Cranial and caudal ends of the tract: ectoderm

2. Intestinal epithelium: endoderm

3. All glands (including liver and pancreas): endoderm

4. Spleen: mesenchymal cells

Questions

1. Which of the following digestive tract malformations is associated with increased MSAFP?

   A. Duodenal atresia
   B. Annular pancreas
   C. Gastroschisis
   D. Meckel's diverticulum
   E. Hirschsprung's disease

2. You are unable to pass a nasogastric tube down on a 2-day-old infant with recurrent vomiting. His x-ray shows presence of air in the stomach. What mechanism is involved in this birth defect?

   A. Failure of recanalization of the esophagus
   B. Deviation of the tracheoesophageal septum
   C. Incomplete recanalization of the esophagus
   D. Failure of recanalization of the duodenum
   E. Failure of neural crest cells to migrate to the wall of the colon

3. The diagram depicted in Figure 46-3 corresponds to an embryo at which stage of development?

   A. Weeks 4 through 6
   B. Weeks 6 through 10
   C. Weeks 11 through 13
   D. Weeks 12 through 14
   E. Weeks 12 through 20

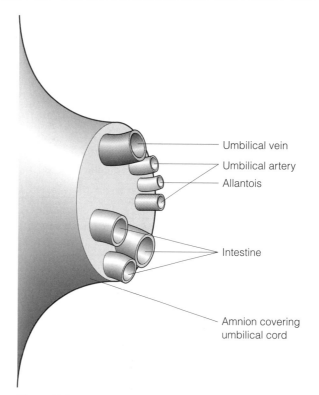

Figure 46-3

HPI: RL is a 33-year-old female at 17 weeks by LMP of her first pregnancy. Today she is having a routine prenatal US. She denies any significant medical history. This pregnancy has been unremarkable so far, and there have been no exposures of concern. Family history (three-generation pedigree) of RL and her husband is noncontributory. The US shows a single living fetus with decreased amniotic fluid (oligohydramnios). The kidneys are not clearly visualized, and the fetal bladder is not seen. The reminder of the fetal anatomy appears normal, although it is technically limited because of the decreased amount of fluid.

PE: Gravid uterus, size less than that estimated by LMP. There is no evidence of amniotic fluid in the vagina on speculum exam, negative ferning, and negative Nitrazine test. A more detailed (level 2) US is performed 2 weeks later at a referral perinatal center. This time, there is absence of amniotic fluid and the kidneys and the bladder are not visualized. The thoracic circumference is small.

Thought Questions

- What is the diagnosis, and what is the etiology?
- What is the natural history of this anomaly?
- What is the developmental error? When did it occur?

Basic Science Review and Discussion

Congenital malformations are the leading cause of infant mortality in the United States. The incidence of major malformations, including mental retardation, in the general population is 3% to 4%.

Bilateral Renal Agenesis   In bilateral renal agenesis a single defect in tissue formation initiates a chain of subsequent defects, which is known as a malformation sequence. The lack of urine will result in decreased and later absent amniotic fluid (oligohydramnios and anhydramnios, respectively). Severe oligohydramnios will result in compression of the fetus, causing limb-positioning defects, abnormal facies (Potter's facies) including beaked nose, small mandible, epicanthic folds, wide-set eyes, and low-set ears. In addition, there is compression of the chest and lack of swallowing of amniotic fluid into the lungs, both of which contribute to pulmonary hypoplasia. This is a uniformly lethal condition, with fetuses either being stillborn or dying shortly after birth from pulmonary hypoplasia.

Abnormalities in the mesonephros may also result in genital malformations (due to failure of the wolffian and müllerian duct to develop or to involute [according to sex]) in about one third of cases of renal agenesis. Other malformations may coexist. The term Potter's syndrome is used to describe bilateral renal agenesis, oligohydramnios, limb deformities, and pulmonary hypoplasia.

Prenatally, the absence of amniotic fluid, an empty bladder, and the lack of kidneys establishes the diagnosis. The etiology is usually unknown, and most cases are sporadic. However, US of the parents or siblings of an affected fetus or newborn is recommended, as 10% of first-degree relatives can have asymptomatic renal malformations (possible AD condition with reduced penetrance and variable expression in some cases).

Embryology   The urogenital system develops from the intermediate mesoderm. Early in the fourth week, during the folding of the embryo, the mesoderm loses connection with the somites and is carried ventrally. A longitudinal elevation or ridge forms on each side of the dorsal aorta, the urogenital ridge, which is composed of the nephrogenic cord, which gives rise to the urinary system and the gonadal ridge, which gives rise to the genital system. Three sets of excretory organs form in the human embryo, the pronephros, the mesonephros, and the metanephros. The pronephros includes rudimentary structures and promptly degenerates, but the pronephric ducts remain and are used by the mesonephros, which appears late in the fourth week caudal to the pronephros. The mesonephros serves as a transient kidney until the permanent kidneys are formed. The mesonephros regresses late in the first trimester; however, their tubules become the efferent ductules of the testes, and the ducts have several adult derivatives in the male. In the fifth week, the metanephros, or permanent kidney, forms and begins making urine at about 9 weeks, mixing in the amniotic cavity. The kidneys form as a result of the metanephric diverticulum or ureteric bud (which is an outgrowth of the mesonephric duct), inducing the formation of the metanephric mass of intermediate mesoderm. Failure of this induction by the ureteric bud results in absence of the kidneys (bilateral renal agenesis). The kidneys are originally placed in the pelvis and gradually ascend as the fetal lumbar and sacral regions grow.

Case Conclusion   After learning the natural history, RL decided to continue with the pregnancy. Four weeks later, she noticed absence of fetal movements, and fetal demise was confirmed by US. Induction of labor was carried out with a PGE_2 analogue. Upon inspection, Potter's facies, dislocation of the hips, and club feet were identified. On autopsy, in addition to the absence of the kidneys, a bicornuate uterus was present. The karyotype was 46,XX. Renal US exams of the parents did not reveal any abnormalities. Two years later, after an uneventful pregnancy, RL delivered a healthy baby girl.

Thumbnail: Renal Development

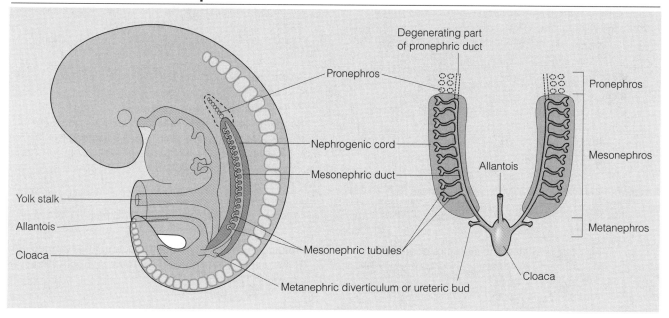

Key Points

▶ Bilateral renal agenesis is characterized by the following:

1. Absence of amniotic fluid
2. Pulmonary hypoplasia
3. Orthopedic deformities
4. Incompatibility with life

Questions

1. Pulmonary hypoplasia and orthopedic deformities can be the result of which of the following?

   A. Diaphragmatic hernia
   B. Prolonged rupture of membranes
   C. Unilateral renal agenesis
   D. Thanatophoric dysplasia
   E. None of the above

2. Prolonged rupture of the fetal membranes and bilateral renal agenesis can have absence of amniotic fluid. You can differentiate between these two conditions antenatally by which of the following?

   A. Karyotype
   B. Detection of amniotic fluid in the vagina
   C. Presence of fetal bladder
   D. B and C are correct
   E. Only autopsy can differentiate between the two conditions

3. In a fetus with bilateral renal agenesis, which of the following is true about the amniotic fluid between 12 and 14 weeks of gestation?

   A. It is absent
   B. Its level is normal
   C. It is decreased
   D. Its level is increased
   E. The level depends on maternal fluid intake

4. A full-term male infant is born with complete exstrophy of the bladder. What is the primary developmental defect?

   A. Incomplete division of the metanephric diverticulum
   B. Internal compression from an ectopic kidney
   C. Complete division of the ureteric bud
   D. Complete patency of the urachus
   E. Failure of mesenchymal cells to migrate between the ectoderm of the abdomen and the cloaca

Answer Key—Part III: Embryology

Case 39

1 A
2 E

Case 40

1 B
2 E
3 E

Case 41

1 C
2 B
3 E

Case 42

1 B
2 C
3 E

Case 43

1 B
2 C
3 E

Case 44

1 B
2 C
3 B

Case 45

1 B
2 A
3 C

Case 46

1 C
2 B
3 B

Case 47

1 B
2 D
3 C
4 E

Answers

Case 1

1. E Each molecule of glucose generates two NADH molecules during glycolysis, two more from the conversion of two molecules of pyruvate to acetyl-CoA, and six more (three each) from the oxidation of acetyl-CoA in the TCA cycle. Of note, the NADH molecules created during glycolysis in the cytosol each generate only two ATP molecules as compared with the three generated by the other NADH molecules in the mitochondria.

2. D Pyruvate dehydrogenase is the enzyme that converts pyruvate to acetyl-CoA. Although its absence or diminished activity can be quite detrimental, it has little effect on erythrocytes, which primarily convert pyruvate to lactate with LDH. Hexokinase, aldolase, and phosphoglycerate kinase are each enzymes in glycolysis that can lead to hemolytic anemia. G6PD deficiency is the most common carbohydrate metabolism enzyme deficiency that can lead to hemolysis. It functions in the pentose phosphate or hexose-monophosphate shunt. This shunt is responsible for regenerating reduced glutathione, which protects the RBCs in the setting of oxidative stress. Thus, patients with G6PD deficiency have a normal hematocrit at baseline but will undergo a hemolytic anemia in the setting of exposure to various conditions including viral or bacterial infections or treatment with drugs such as antimalarials, sulfonamides, and nitrofurantoin.

Case 2

1. D Because of their hindered ability to produce fatty acids, individuals with diminished pyruvate dehydrogenase activity often have decreased myelination. Multiple fractures might be seen in patients with osteogenesis imperfecta, a collagen synthesis disorder. An enlarged liver would be seen in patients with glycogen storage diseases. A lateral neck cyst is often the result of failure of the branchial arches to entirely close and is called a *branchial arch cyst*. A cardiac VSD is associated with a number of syndromes, but pyruvate dehydrogenase deficiency is not one of them.

2. D If acetyl-CoA could not enter the TCA cycle, the principal problem would be a matter of diminished production of energy from each molecule of glucose. Thus, there would need to be increased glycolysis and metabolism of ketoacids. As a result, there would be a minimal increase in acetyl-CoA levels (because the acetyl-CoA molecules would be used in these synthetic pathways, too). We would not see decreased myelination, fractures, or an enlarged liver, as discussed previously. There would likely be an increased level of oxaloacetate because it is the molecule that combines with acetyl-CoA and is synthesized from acetyl-CoA.

Case 3

1. B With any of the enzymes specific to gluconeogenesis being deficient, one would expect there to be less glucose, but elevated levels of pyruvate, lactate, and acetyl-CoA. In enzyme deficiencies of the initial enzymes, pyruvate carboxylase, and PEP carboxykinase, one would expect these deviations to be greater. In this case, because these two enzymes are normal, there is likely to be an elevation in oxaloacetate as well. Because the enzyme in question, fructose-1,6-bisphosphatase, uses fructose-1,6-diphosphate, that molecule is likely to be slightly elevated, although it can be reversibly metabolized back through glycolysis.

2. A Phosphoglucose isomerase converts G6P and fructose-6-phosphate back and forth. Hexokinase, pyruvate kinase, and phosphofructokinase all catalyze irreversible reactions in glycolysis while G6Pase catalyzes an irreversible reaction in gluconeogenesis.

3. B Thiamine is a cofactor for the pyruvate dehydrogenase complex, which converts pyruvate to acetyl-CoA. By supplementing the diet with thiamine, there is a hope to decrease levels of pyruvate and lactate, which lessens the accompanying metabolic acidosis. It would not help with the decreased glucose levels, and it would not have an impact on glycogen synthesis or liver size. Myelination is not deficient in pyruvate carboxylase deficiency, because acetyl-CoA levels and fatty acid production are normal to increased.

Case 4

1. B The glycogen storage diseases can be broken into several categories. One is those diseases leading to hepatic hypoglycemic pathophysiology. Of these, there are the varieties of type I, which have elevated levels of G6P and its metabolites, and types III (Cori), VI (Hers'), and VIII in which G6P levels are usually diminished. In this case, because of the increased serum lactate level, there is a good chance that this is a variety of type I disease. However, with the normal level of G6Pase, it is not von Gierke's disease. The second most common cause of type I disease is G6P microsomal translocase deficiency, which leaves the hepatic tissue without the ability to transport G6P into the endoplasmic reticulum and eventually convert to glucose and be transported out of the cell. The increased lactate essentially rules out Cori's and Hers' disease. McArdle's disease is one of diminished muscle capacity.

2. E, 3. C Another group of the glycogen storage diseases includes those that specifically affect the muscles. These include type V (McArdle's) and several varieties of type VII. These diseases usually present between ages 10 and 30 with painful cramps, muscle weakness, and myoglobinuria. They can be diagnosed by muscle biopsy and assessment of enzyme activity. In McArdle's disease, which is an AR disorder mapped to chromosome 11, the inactive enzyme is muscle glycogen phosphorylase. The enzyme deficiencies in type VII include phosphofructokinase and phosphoglycerate mutase. Treatment of these diseases includes avoidance of vigorous activity and ingesting glucose before exercise. See the following table for how these diseases commonly present.

Glycogen storage disease	Enzyme deficiency	Presentation	Prognosis/Rx
Type IA—von Gierke	Glucose-6-phosphatase	Hypoglycemia by age 12 mo	Developmental delay; renal failure (dietary Rx)
Type IB	G6P microsomal translocase	Hypoglycemia by age 12 mo	Similar to IA plus neutropenia, recurrent infections
Type II—Pompe	α-1,4-glucosidase	Weakness, cardiomegaly	Death by age 2 or 3 yr
Type III—Cori	Debranching enzyme	Hepatomegaly, hypoglycemia	Dietary Rx
Type IV—Andersen	Branching enzyme	Hypotonia as infant, cirrhosis	Death by age 2 or 3 yr
Type V—McArdle	Glycogen phosphorylase (muscle)	Cramps and pain after exercise	Avoid exercise, prefeed
Type VI—Hers' disease	Glycogen phosphorylase (liver)	Hepatomegaly, mild hypoglycemia	Dietary Rx
Type VII	Phosphofructokinase (muscle)	Cramps and pain after exercise	Avoid exercise, mild anemia, prefeed
Type VIII	Phosphorylase kinase (liver)	Hepatomegaly, mild hypoglycemia	Dietary Rx

Case 5

1. D The α-glycerol phosphate shuttle produces $FADH_2$ in the mitochondria rather than NADH produced by the malate shuttle. Thus, there are two as compared to three ATP molecules produced per NADH molecule from the cytosol. The conversion of pyruvate to acetyl-CoA results in production of 1 NADH molecule, and a turn of the citric acid cycle produces 3 NADH, 1 GTP, and 1 $FADH_2$ molecule, all in the mitochondria, so the net result is 15 ATP produced. When added to the four produced via the $FADH_2$ from the α-glycerol phosphate shuttle, this makes a total of 19.

2. A Mitochondria and therefore mtDNA are only inherited maternally because the ovum is the sole source of mitochondria. Because LA is male, his children have no chance of being affected as long as their mother is not affected.

3. E There are two NADH and two ATP molecules produced by glycolysis in the cytosol. There are also two pyruvate molecules formed, which rapidly pass into the mitochondria. As in question 1, each pyruvate molecule generates 15 ATP. Because the two NADH molecules in the cytosol cannot enter the mitochondria without a shuttle, the net total ATP production is 32.

Case 6

1. C The carnitine diet supplementation can help provide carnitine as a substrate for CAT-I to transport fatty acids into the mitochondria. Because the very short fatty acid chains and the long-chain fatty acids can undergo some β-oxidation, yielding a fuel source of acetyl-CoA molecules, carnitine's effect is to increase the transport of the activated fatty acids across the mitochondrial membrane. The body acts carnitine deficient despite having elevated total levels, because the carnitine molecules remain bound to CAT-II in the mitochondria. Carnitine does not influence the enzyme listed, and although an effort was to increase acetyl-CoA levels, carnitine cannot enter the TCA cycle at a later point.

2. A Hardy-Weinberg equilibrium uses $p^2 + 2pq + q^2 = 1$. Because the homozygous recessive rate in that population was 0.81, the

prevalence of the mutation K304E is 0.9. If $p = .9$, then $q = .1$, or 10%. Nine is the percentage of non-K304E mutations. Heterozygotes would number 2pq, or 18%. This leads the other homozygous population to be 1%, or .01.

3. B Insulin and glucagon do much to maintain homeostasis. In general, glucagon leads to increased levels of fuel for tissues, and thus breakdown of fats and glycogen and increases in glucose levels. Insulin does the opposite, leading to storage of carbohydrates and fatty acids. So, of the four changes, only a decrease in CAT-I activity would lead to more storage. CAT-I and CAT-II are responsible for getting fatty acids into mitochondria so they can be oxidized. Fatty acyl-CoA synthetase activates fatty acids, so an increase would also lead to oxidation. Fatty acyl-CoA carboxylase is an enzyme in the fatty acid synthesis pathway, and thus would be increased by insulin. Protein catabolism would be stimulated by glucagon, not insulin.

Case 7

1. E If the 11β-hydroxylase enzyme is absent, the patient does experience CAH, but in this case because it is a male infant, there will not be any obvious phenotypic changes, and usually presentation is with failure to thrive. In CAH, cholesterol and pregnenolone levels are usually relatively normal. The immediate substrates of 11β-hydroxylase, 11-deoxycortisol, and 11-deoxycorticosterone would be elevated, as would androstenedione and often testosterone. However, in this male infant, without aromatase enzyme, estrone would not be elevated.

2. C CAH is a constellation of absence of glucocorticoids, often mineralocorticoids, buildup of precursors and androgens, and the phenotypic response to these hormonal changes. 3β-Hydroxysteroid dehydrogenase deficiency is the third most common cause of CAH. If the C20,22-desmolase was missing, cholesterol would not be able to proceed down the common pathway, and none of the steroid hormones would be synthesized. If C17,20-desmolase was missing, the androgens would not be synthesized, but the other steroid hormones would undergo normal synthesis. If the 18-hydroxy enzymes were missing, aldosterone synthesis would not occur, but cortisol would still be synthesized.

Case 8

1. A Patients with SLO syndrome have an enzymatic defect in the enzyme DHCR7, which takes 7DHC into cholesterol. Thus, these patients have elevated levels of 7DHC. A patient on enormously high quantities of HMG-CoA reductase inhibitors would have increased levels of HMG-CoA, the molecule that is reduced, and decreased levels of mevalonate, the product of this enzymatic reaction, as compared with normal patients. They would also have decreased levels of all of the molecules downstream (such as 7DHC and cholesterol). Patients with SLO syndrome are likely to have normal or high levels of these molecules because they have an enzymatic block in this pathway much further downstream.

2. C HMG-CoA to mevalonate, the rate-limiting step of cholesterol synthesis, is catalyzed by HMG-CoA reductase. This is the key site of regulation and a target for cholesterol-lowering agents. The first two steps (A and B) are not important regulatory steps. Mevalonate to isopentenyl pyrophosphate actually takes several steps and requires three ATP molecules. 7DHC to cholesterol is the step that does not occur in patients with SLO syndrome.

Case 9

1. A Lipoprotein lipase primarily hydrolyzes triacylglycerols in either chylomicrons or VLDLs. This hydrolysis results in an increase in the percentage weight of these molecules, converting into VLDLs, LDLs, HDLs, and so on. Chylomicrons do get converted into VLDLs, but it is rare for HDL to be an end product. Apo B-100 facilitates the production of VLDLs by providing respite from the weary, but an increase in weather, depending on overkill.

2. B All of these patients are at risk of developing cardiovascular disease, but only one fits the description in the question. The patient with lipoprotein lipase deficiency will have relatively normal or even low levels of LDL and VLDL, because the enzyme normally helps produce these molecules, particularly from chylomicrons. The other two genetic-risk patients will have elevated LDLs and VLDLs. The other at-risk patients would be likely to have increased LDLs and VLDLs as well with the smoking and obesity histories and would not be at particular risk of having xanthomas.

Case 10

1. D The etiology of preeclampsia is not fully understood. Likely involved is an imbalance of thromboxane/prostacyclin as a result of deficient intravascular production of prostacyclin (vasodilation) and excessive production of thromboxane (favoring vasoconstriction and platelet aggregation). These observations have led to the hypothesis that antiplatelet agents (low-dose aspirin) might prevent or delay the onset of preeclampsia.

2. C Aspirin and NSAIDs, such as indomethacin, ibuprofen, and COX inhibitors, inhibit COX, and therefore inhibit prostaglandin synthesis. Glucocorticoids are powerful anti-inflammatory agents, which act to inhibit the release of AA from membrane phospholipids. Glucocorticoids affect both the COX and the lipoxygenase pathway and therefore inhibit the production of leukotrienes and prostaglandins. (See Figure 10-1.)

Case 11

1. A There is significant overlap in the phenotype of **Marfan's syndrome** and homocystinuria. Both disorders have similar musculoskeletal and ocular findings. Cardiac manifestations are one of the hallmarks of Marfan's (mitral valve prolapse, aortic dilation) but are not part of homocystinuria. In addition, mental retardation and thromboembolic complications are *not* typical features of Marfan's syndrome. The sudden onset of severe chest pain in a patient with the phenotype described suggests dissection of the aorta in a patient with Marfan's syndrome. Marfan's syndrome is caused by mutations in the **fibrillin-1 gene.** CBS deficiency is the enzymatic defect responsible for homocystinuria. Patients with homozygosity of MTHFR mutation variants may have mild elevations of homocysteine and are at an increased risk of vascular complications but do not have a distinct phenotype and are not at increased risk of aortic dilation/dissection.

2. A Mild elevations of homocysteine have been associated with common medical problems, including vascular disease in the coronary, carotid and peripheral circulations, increased risk of dementia, increased risk of NTDs, and possibly cleft lip and palate. The mechanism by which this occurs is not fully understood. Proposed mechanisms include oxidative injury to the vascular wall, vascular cell proliferation, and development of a prothrombotic state. The elevations of homocysteine may be the result of vitamin or cofactor deficiency in the homocysteine pathway, genetically determined (as in MTHFR homozygote variants), or a combination of genetic and environmental interactions. Protein C deficiency and factor V Leiden mutations are procoagulant conditions but are not associated with elevated homocysteine. Dolichostenomelia (tall, slender) and mental retardation are in keeping with homocystinuria, which has elevated, *not* normal, levels of methionine. Holoprosencephaly is genetically heterogeneous but is not associated with homocysteine elevations.

3. E For those children with homocystinuria not identified through newborn screening, the diagnosis may be first suspected between 3 and 5 years of age when ocular manifestations become apparent. The mental retardation is progressive if untreated. Some musculoskeletal findings might be present but become more apparent with age. **Cyanide nitroprusside test** is used as a screening test in some **newborn screening** programs. The metabolic abnormality consists of elevations of homocysteine and methionine and low or absent cysteine. The diagnosis is confirmed by decreased or absent CBS activity. Hyperphenylalaninemia is the hallmark of PKU, the most common IEM associated with mental retardation, if left untreated.

Case 12

1. B Females with PKU who are not on a strict phenylalanine-restricted diet are at risk of having children who are mentally retarded, microcephalic, growth restricted, and have a high incidence of congenital heart defects. This phenotype is directly related to the levels of phenylalanine in the maternal blood and not related to the fetal genotype. It is essential that females with PKU remain in contact with a metabolic facility, are offered effective means of contraception, and receive optimal preconceptional treatment. With adequate dietary treatment, evidenced by phenylalanine and tyrosine levels within the normal range, the outcome in offspring of mothers with PKU should be the same as that of controls.

2. D For nuclear families in which there is an affected individual with PKU and both parents are available, it is possible to offer linkage analysis and predict whether the fetus carries the defective haplotypes by either CVS or amniocentesis. Though possible to do a fetal liver biopsy and test for PAH activity, it is a procedure that carries significant risk to the fetus. PAH activity is not expressed in amniocytes. DNA testing is not possible because we know that mutation analysis failed to identify one mutation in the affected (homozygous) son.

3. C *Galactosemia* is due to a deficiency of **galactose-1-uridyltransferase** (GALT). The neonatal presentation with liver failure and *Escherichia coli* sepsis is classic. Infants who survive develop mental retardation, chronic liver failure, and cataracts. Females will develop ovarian failure. Treatment consists of removal of all galactose from the diet.

Tyrosinemia I is characterized by liver dysfunction, liver failure, and cirrhosis but is not associated with cataracts. The defect is due to a deficiency in the distal pathway of tyrosine catabolism, leading to accumulation of succinylacetone, the hallmark of this disorder. **Homocystinuria** due to CBS deficiency is characterized by mental retardation, skeletal abnormalities, ectopia lentis, and a tendency for thromboembolism. **Biotinidase deficiency** can be successfully treated with large doses of biotin and will not lead to the serious neurologic symptoms (seizures, mental retardation, hearing loss, and hypotonia) seen in untreated patients. All of these disorders are AR IEMs that are currently screened in most newborn screening programs.

Case 13

1. C Ascorbic acid is needed as a reducing agent to maintain the iron atom in prolyl hydroxylase in the ferrous state, thereby keeping it in an active state. In the absence of a reducing agent and functional prolyl hydroxylase, the collagen synthesized becomes insufficiently hydroxylated and the triple helix is much less stable. This abnormal collagen has a lower melting temperature and cannot appropriately form fibers. Scurvy, which is caused by a dietary insufficiency of ascorbic acid, is characterized by skin lesions, poor healing, hypertrophic bleeding gums, and easy bruising due to fragile blood vessels.

2. C The missense mutation in the proα1(I) is an example of dominant negative alleles where a mutant allele can lead to a dominant phenotype because of the polymeric nature of the final protein. In type I OI, a mutation leading to an absence of gene product (proα1^0 null allele) has a milder phenotype because overall the collagen formed is normal but just reduced in number. The other mutations listed are causes of other types of OI.

3. D Collagen is unique for many reasons. It has a very regular sequence of glycine-proline-hydroxyproline. In contrast, globular-type proteins rarely have any regularity in their sequence. Also, the proportion of glycine is much higher and it is seen almost at every third position. Glycine plays a critical role in the helical nature of collagen because it is small enough to fit in the interior position of the helix, and because it occupies very little space, it allows different polypeptide strands to come together. Proline is also found in higher concentrations in collagen than in other proteins. However, it is not found in nearly every third position as with glycine. In addition, the presence of hydroxylysine and hydroxyproline is unique because it is rarely found in other proteins. They are incorporated first as lysine and proline into procollagen, and only a small proportion of these residues are hydroxylated in a highly specific manner.

Case 14

1. D Each purine ring is created from a variety of precursors and includes glutamine, aspartate, glycine, MTHF, N^{10}-formyltetrahydrofolate, and CO_2. The purine ring is formed on a ribose phosphate, which is a product of the pentose phosphate pathway. Carbamoylphosphate is a precursor to the pyrimidine nucleotides.

2. D The pentose phosphate pathway generates NADPH and ribose 5-phosphate in the cytosol. This ribose 5-phosphate is the backbone structure in the formation of both purines and pyrimidines. The urea cycle is important in the degradation of amino acids. Glycolysis is a series of reactions converting glucose into pyruvate with the concomitant production of ATP. Gluconeogenesis is the synthesis of glucose from noncarbohydrate sources, such as lactate, amino acids, and glycerol. The citric acid cycle is a series of reactions that serve as the final common pathway for the oxidation of fuel molecules, as well as a source of intermediate molecules in multiple biosynthetic pathways.

3. A Both purine and pyrimidine synthesis are regulated by feedback inhibition.

4. A The patient in this scenario has gout. Gout results most commonly from an increase in uric acid either because of decreased renal clearance or increased production or destruction of purines. The increased uric acid can lead to the precipitation of sodium urate crystals. Commonly, these crystals are deposited in the joints and kidneys, causing renal dysfunction and extreme pain. Treatment of gout is initially by pain control, and over time, the crystals are diminished by allopurinol. This drug is metabolized to alloxantin, which stays bound to the active site of xanthine oxidase. This decreases production of uric acid and leads to crystal dissolution.

Case 15

1. B Homozygosity for PBG deficiency, the rate-limiting enzyme in AIP, is rare but results in severely affected individuals. If both parents are carriers of the mutant gene, they have a 25% chance of having a homozygous child, 50% of heterozygous, and 25% chance of not being a carrier. Is important to note that only 10%

of known carriers of PBG deficiency are manifesting heterozygotes. Although usually rare, there are many examples of homozygosity of AD disorders, usually leading to a severe phenotype, often not compatible with life, such as in achondroplasia, the most common form of inherited dwarfism.

2. D It is well known that a large group of medications can exacerbate or precipitate an acute episode of porphyria. Always before prescribing a medication, the physician must check this list in a patient known to have porphyria. The mechanism by which this occurs is by induction of the earlier rate-controlling step in heme synthesis, δ-aminolevulinic acid synthesis. **Barbiturates, sulfonamides, and anticonvulsants are the usual examples given.** Because seizures may occur in AIP, the choice of anticonvulsants is important. Phenytoin is probably the least toxic anticonvulsant in the setting of AIP. The other medications listed are commonly used in the treatment of acute episodes of AIP, with the exception of ibuprofen, which is typically not effective in the control of the severe pain of these patients.

Case 16

1. A From the text in this case, we know that short-term regulation of the cycle occurs principally at CPS-I, which is relatively inactive in the absence of its allosteric activator N-acetylglutamate. The steady-state concentration of N-acetylglutamate is set by the concentration of its components acetyl-CoA and glutamate and by arginine, which is a positive allosteric effector of N-acetylglutamate synthetase. The other enzymes are from the urea cycle, but they are minimally involved in the regulation of the cycle.

2. C IEMs can cause symptoms in two primary ways, not making enough of something or not breaking down or clearing a molecule. In patients with UCDs, what they have in common is the decreased ability to break down and excrete the nitrogenous waste from proteins and amino acids. This leads to a buildup of ammonia, which leads to the neurologic and mental status changes seen in patients with UCDs. These patients clear urea and orotic acid relatively quickly via renal excretion, so although orotic acid may be slightly elevated in OTC-deficient patients, it is not thought to be a cause of their symptoms. Urea is actually decreased, not elevated. There is no particular change in renal function in these patients.

Case 17

1. C Insulin stimulates anabolic processes and inhibits catabolic processes. The downstream effects of insulin signaling include gene expression, growth regulation, glucose utilization, and synthesis of glycogen, lipid, and proteins. It promotes the uptake of glucose, other sugars, and amino acids into muscle and fat cells. It also functions to decrease gluconeogenesis, by lowering the level of enzymes such as pyruvate carboxylase and fructose-1,6-bisphosphatase.

2. C Protein kinase A phosphorylates serine and threonine residues on the insulin receptor, causing a decrease in tyrosine kinase activity. A decrease in insulin receptor activity would not result in an

increase in autophosphorylation of the receptor and would not result in an increase in receptor phosphorylation of tyrosine residues of downstream targets. Decreases in receptor activity would cause a decrease in the synthesis of glycogen. Inhibition of insulin receptor activity would not affect protein kinase C through this pathway. In addition, inhibition of receptor activity would not decrease insulin production by the β-cells but may increase production of insulin in cases in which the β-cells are still able to produce insulin and there is an elevated serum glucose level.

Case 18

1. A TCRs are specific for the combination of a peptide and the MHC protein presenting the peptide (MHC restriction). They do not recognize an isolated foreign molecule. TCRs are found membrane bound, whereas immunoglobulins can be either secreted or membrane bound. The peptides that are presented and recognized by a TCR are typically less than 10 amino acids in length. They are processed to this length in the lysosomes of the antigen-presenting cells. The diversity of TCRs is due to the recombination of V, D, J segments, the imprecision at the junctions, and the different α/β or γ/δ combinations. The α, β, γ, and δ chains do not form pairs by a combination of any of the 4 chains, but specifically α/β or γ/δ. Superantigens cause illness by the nonspecific stimulation of T-cells through a common V_β, resulting in the secretion of large amounts of cytokines.

2. B Superantigens cause illness by the nonspecific stimulation of T-cells through a common V_β, resulting in the secretion of large amounts of cytokines. Superantigens bind to the side of the MHC protein, which is on the antigen-presenting cell, and the V_β of the TCR.

3. C Class II proteins encode the HLA antigens and are highly polymorphic, not conserved. HLA antigens have been associated with different diseases. Most of the diseases are autoimmune diseases such as ankylosing spondylitis, celiac disease, type I diabetes, rheumatoid arthritis, multiple sclerosis, myasthenia gravis, and SLE. The class I proteins are composed of an α chain and β_2-microglobulin and play an integral role in antigen presentation, not in the complement cascade. Class I and II proteins, not class II and III proteins, bind peptide and are integral in antigen presentation. Class I and II proteins, TCRs, immunoglobulins, and some growth factors and molecules in the nervous system all share some homology, placing them in the immunoglobulin superfamily. The class III, however, are not included.

Case 19

1. C Epinephrine stimulation of its cognate receptor results in activation of the G-protein, activation of adenylate cyclase, production of cAMP, and activation of downstream kinases by cAMP. In the case of protein kinase A, the binding of cAMP to the regulatory subunits results in the release of the catalytic subunits, which then become enzymatically active. Phosphorylation of the C-terminus end of the hormone receptor regulates this pathway with phosphorylation typically preventing receptor activation of the downstream G-protein. G$_i$ negatively regulates the activity of G$_s$ by the β/γ subunits from G$_i$ binding to G$_s$ to cause a reversal in the activation of adenylate cyclase. The intrinsic GTPase activity of the α subunit negatively regulates this pathway by slowly converting the active GTP form into the inactive GDP form. ADP ribosylation of G$_s$ is not a form of regulation for this pathway but is the cause of disease in pertussis and cholera.

2. C Pertussis toxin catalyzes the addition of an ADP ribose to a specific cysteine side chain on the α subunit of G$_i$, fixing it in the inactive GDP form. GTP is unable to bind and cause the dissociation of β/γ that is needed for it to bind to G$_s$. Therefore, G$_i$ is unable to negatively regulate adenylate cyclase and cAMP is continually produced. cAMP is then available to activate protein kinase A and causes other downstream effects. The phospholipase C and phosphoinositide signaling pathway is coupled to a different G-protein, G$_{PLC}$, which is stimulated by the mast cell IgE receptor and a chemotactic receptor. This pathway can also be activated by pertussis toxin. Stimulation of this pathway by hormone-receptor interaction leads to activation of phospholipase C, a membrane-bound enzyme, the hydrolysis of PIP$_2$ to give two molecules involved in signaling: inositol 1,4,5-triphosphate (IP$_3$) and diacylglycerol (DAG). The GTPase activity is not a target of the pertussis toxin.

Case 20

1. B This patient has both pernicious anemia and the neurologic symptoms that accompany vitamin B$_{12}$ deficiency. These neurologic symptoms begin as paresthesias, progressing to an awkward unsteady gait and eventually stiffness of the limbs. These symptoms are related to demyelination of the nerves. If vitamin B$_{12}$ supplementation is begun within a week or two of symptoms, there may be complete resolution of disease, although with a prolonged presence of symptoms, recovery may be only minimal. Folate (not listed) can also cause a macrocytic anemia. Thiamine (vitamin B$_1$) deficiency, as in the case, can cause neurologic symptoms, but the presentation is different from this.

2. C Deficiency in vitamin C leads to **scurvy** because of the role of the vitamin in the post-translational modification of collagens. Scurvy is characterized by easily bruised skin, muscle fatigue, soft swollen gums, decreased wound healing and hemorrhaging, osteoporosis, and anemia. Vitamin C is readily absorbed, and thus the primary cause of vitamin C deficiency is poor diet and/or an increased requirement. Classically, scurvy was seen on long sea voyages when citrus fruit was not available. The osteoporosis in this case may have led to a diagnosis of vitamin D deficiency. However, rickets and osteomalacia do not present with decreased healing.

Case 21

1. D Because both parents are carriers, they have a 25% chance of having an unaffected child. The chance of having two unaffected children is 0.25 × 0.25, or 6.25%.

2. B In both disorders, affected mothers have a 50% chance of transmitting the disease to their children. In X-linked disorders, females are affected twice as commonly as males. One of the characteristic features of AD diseases is male-to-male transmission, which is not seen in X-linked disorders. Skipped generations are not seen in either AD or X-linked dominant pedigrees. In AD traits, affected males have a 50% chance of passing the diseased allele to both their sons and their daughters.

3. C This patient has Huntington's disease, an AD disorder caused by expanding CAG trinucleotide repeats in the Huntington gene. Characteristic features of this disorder include involuntary twitching movements (chorea) and progressive loss of voluntary muscle control. Depression, dementia, and other psychiatric symptoms are common in patients with Huntington's disease.

4. C The above protocol describes the Southern blot technique and is used in the diagnosis of myotonic dystrophy. PCR involves the amplification of a specific DNA sequence. Western blot is a technique in which protein is run through a gel, transferred to a membrane, and then hybridized with labeled antibodies. This test is used for the diagnosis of diseases such as HIV and Lyme disease. FISH is a procedure in which fluorescence-labeled probes are hybridized with chromosomes and then visualized with a fluorescence microscope. Northern blot is similar to the Southern blot, except that RNA is run through the gel instead of DNA.

Case 22

1. B The gene product of the **CF** gene or CFTR protein is believed to participate in chloride transport and mucin secretion. The protein has a complex three-dimensional structure, with two transmembrane (TM) domains, which anchor it to the cell membrane, two nucleotide-binding folds (NBFs), which bind ATP, and a regulatory (R) domain, which has several phosphorylation sites.

2. B In AR disorders, if each parent has one mutant allele, the chances of an affected offspring is 1 in 4, to be a carrier 1 in 2, and to not be a carrier is 1 in 4, according to Mendel's law. However, in the case presented, the sister is not affected, so she can only be a carrier (2/3 chance) or not a carrier (1/3 chance). Because the husband has not been screened, we must use the known carrier frequency for that population (1/25). The chance that the mutant allele is passed on is 1 in 2 for each parent. So then the equation is: 2/3 * 1/2 * 1/25 * 1/2 = 1/150, or 1 in 150.

3. D Nonpaternity or "false paternity" may be as common as 15% in certain populations. Genetic testing may incidentally disclose nonpaternity in the work-up of a genetic disorder of an affected offspring. This issue must be addressed in the counseling before testing. Commercially available DNA panels screen only for the more common mutations (usually 32 to 72 for patients with CF), but there are more than 400 known mutations. This is particularly important among certain ethnic groups in which CF is rare and a large proportion of the mutations are unknown (for example Hispanics and Asians). In AR disorders heterozygous (carriers) are by definition not affected.

Case 23

1. C Because WL's mother is a known carrier, his maternal grandmother must also have been a carrier because neither parent has muscular dystrophy. Therefore, the aunt has a 50% chance of inheriting the mutated allele from WL's grandmother.

2. C The mother and father both have one abnormal X chromosome. WL's daughter will inherit a diseased allele from her father and will have a 50% chance of inheriting a normal allele from her mother. Therefore, she has a 50% chance of being a carrier and a 50% chance of being affected. If the parents have a son, he would have a 50% chance of being normal and a 50% chance of having the disease trait.

3. A An affected male is unable to pass an X-linked mutation to his son. So even if WL's grandfather does have the dystrophin deletion, his grandmother must still be a carrier because their son is affected.

4. D This clinical scenario is characteristic of hemophilia A, an X-linked recessive disorder. This disease is caused by deficient or abnormal clotting factor VIII and results in frequent bruising, prolonged bleeding from wounds, and hemorrhage into joints. Treatment is with factor VIII infusions. Hemophilia B is an X-linked disorder characterized by deficient clotting factor IX. It is less common and less severe than hemophilia A. A third major bleeding disorder is von Willebrand's disease, an AD disorder caused by deficient carrier protein for factor VIII. Platelet activity is normal in hemophilia and von Willebrand's diseases.

Case 24

1. C TR's sister has a 50% chance of having the full mutation and 50% chance of having a normal allele (she cannot be a premutation carrier because it almost always expands when the mother has a premutation in the more than 90-repeat range). She has a 50% chance of transmitting the mutant allele to each of her daughters who have a 50% chance of being mentally retarded (affected) if they inherited the mutation. So the risk is 1/2 * 1/2 * 1/2 = 1 in 8 chance (the risk of having a mentally retarded son would be 1 in 4 because all males with the full mutation are mentally retarded).

2. D TR's uncle is a premutation carrier, so neither he nor his children are affected. Because the mutant allele is in the X chromosome, he cannot pass the premutation to his son. All daughters of premutation carrier fathers will inherit the premutation unchanged (stable) or with mild expansion (but still in the premutation range) and hence be unaffected. The premutation daughter can then transmit and have an expansion of repeats to the next generation to 50% of sons and daughters. If the mutation expanded to the full mutation range (>200), all males will be affected and roughly one half of the females will be affected.

3. A Unstable or dynamic mutations caused by triplet repeat sequences of DNA can expand over the course of generations, explaining complex inheritance patterns (such as for Fragile X or myotonic dystrophy) that were largely unexplained until recently. Some AD disorders exhibit earlier disease onset in the offspring than the parents and increasing disease severity in subsequent generations. This phenomenon, known as *anticipation,* is well established in **myotonic dystrophy** and **Huntington's disease,** which are both examples of AD unstable expansion triplet repeat DNA sequences. In myotonic dystrophy, an expansion of a CTG triplet repeat can account for the severe neonatal presentation of myotonic dystrophy, which occurs only when the mutation is inherited from the mother. In Huntington's disease, an expansion of a CAG triplet repeat can account for the juvenile form of the disease when the mutation is passed on by the father. The cause for this sex bias in anticipation is unclear.

Case 25

1. D Males with a mitochondrial disorder cannot pass on the mutation, whereas males with an X-linked recessive mutation can only produce either a normal son or a carrier female. So assuming that the female has normal genotype, no offspring of a male with either a mitochondrial or an X-linked recessive disorder will be affected. In X-linked disorders, both the male and the female can pass the mutation on to the next generation. In mitochondrial inheritance, males and females are affected at an equal rate, but it is only the female who can transmit the mutation. A mother with an X-linked recessive disorder will have affected sons but asymptomatic daughters.

2. A A female with a mitochondrial mutation will transmit the mutation to all of her children. Because we know that the affected individual's mother has the mutation, all of the maternal aunts must also have the mutation.

3. B Heteroplasmy defines the ability of a cell to have multiple species of mtDNA. The threshold effect describes the phenomenon of when symptoms are manifested only after a certain level of mutant mtDNA has been reached. Homoplasmy occurs when a cell has only one population of mtDNA. Pleiotropy is the ability of a gene to direct more than one phenotype. Imprinting is the concept that differences in phenotype occur depending on whether a genetic mutation is inherited from the mother or the father.

Case 26

1. D Variable expression is the concept that the severity of a genetic disease can be modified by the environment, allelic heterogeneity, or modifier genes. Reduced penetrance occurs when an individual has a disease gene, but not the disease phenotype. This is an all-or-nothing phenomenon. Imprinting is the variable phenotype of a genetic mutation depending on the parental origin of the disease gene. Pleiotropy defines the ability of a gene to influence multiple phenotypes. Anticipation refers to the earlier expression and increasing severity of a disease phenotype with successive generations.

2. E This family has features characteristic of tuberous sclerosis. Tuberous sclerosis is an AD disease with highly variable expressivity, even among family members, and is the second most common neurocutaneous syndrome (the first being NF1). Manifestations of Sturge-Weber syndrome include congenital, unilateral capillary angiomas of the head and neck, as well as seizures. NF2 is also an AD disease characterized by eighth nerve tumors and is frequently associated with other intracranial or intraspinal tumors. Von Recklinghausen is the German pathologist who first described the constellation of symptoms in NF and his name is now synonymous for NF1. Marfan's syndrome is an AD disorder with a defect in the connective tissue protein **fibrillin.** Characteristic defects are seen in the ocular (detached lens), skeletal (long, slender limbs, and fingers), and cardiovascular (mitral valve prolapse, aortic aneurysm) systems.

3. C Locus heterogeneity is the ability of mutations in different genes to cause the same disease phenotype. Pleiotropy describes genes that can cause multiple phenotypes. Allelic heterogeneity is defined as the variation in disease phenotype depending on the type or location of mutations in a disease gene. Heteroplasmy is seen in mitochondrial genetics and is the presence of multiple species of DNA at a particular locus within a cell. When there are individuals in a population who have a disease genotype, but not the disease phenotype, the disease genotype is said to have reduced or incomplete penetrance.

Case 27

1. C The thought is that Tay-Sachs occurs so frequently in the Ashkenazi Jewish population because of either the founder effect, where the high frequency of a mutant gene in a population is founded by a small ancestral group when one or more founders is a carrier for the mutation, or a heterozygote advantage, where being heterozygote for the mutation offers a selection advantage over both homozygous genotypes. When a recessive trait is high in a population, consanguinity is not the cause of an affected child. Consanguinity is a cause when the recessive carrier rate is low. Tay-Sachs is an AR disorder resulting from a single-gene mutation in the α subunit locus. Sandhoff's disease and activator deficiency occurs when a mutation exists in the β subunit or in the activator protein, respectively.

2. D There are multiple single-gene mutations that lead to the disease, but there are two common ones. The first involves a 4-bp insertion into exon 11, resulting in a premature stop codon. The second mutation is an error in RNA splicing in exon 12 that results in a substitution of a cytosine in place of a guanine, and splicing does not occur. An inversion is when a single chromosome undergoes two breaks and is reconstituted with the segment between the breaks in an inverted position. Recombination error is mutation that results from a combination of linked genes on homologous chromosomes during a crossover of their loci. Translocations can cause mutations when there is an exchange of chromosome segments between nonhomologous chromosomes resulting in an abnormal product. Gene deletion is a loss of a gene or part of a gene from a chromosome.

3. D Tay-Sachs is due to the deficiency of Hex A, the enzyme responsible for the degradation of G_{M2} gangliosides. G_{M2} ganglio-

side is what becomes accumulated in neurons in Tay-Sachs. Sphingomyelinase deficiency is seen in Niemann-Pick disease. Glucocerebroside deficiency is seen in Gaucher's disease. Arylsulfatase A deficiency causes metachromatic leukodystrophy.

Case 28

1. B For couples who have had one prior affected offspring with trisomy 21, the empiric recurrence risk is 1% greater than that expected for age-specific risk. This high incidence (particularly for younger couples) can be explained by trisomy 21 **gonadal mosaicism.** In 3% of DS, the extra chromosome 21 is fused with another acrocentric chromosome, known as a **robertsonian translocation.** The parents of translocation DS children need to be karyotyped because one third of the time, one of the parents will be a **balance translocation carrier.** These individuals are at a particularly high risk of recurrence of DS and for spontaneous abortion, which, depending on the translocation and the parent carrying it, can be as high as 100%.

2. B Because a high proportion of trisomy 21 (30%) are spontaneously lost, earlier detection by **CVS** detects a proportion of cases that would not have been picked up by a later procedure. This phenomenon is true for the other chromosomal aneuploidies as well. CVS is generally performed between 10 and 13 weeks of gestation. Its main advantage over amniocentesis is earlier diagnosis. The disadvantages of CVS over amniocentesis are a higher pregnancy loss rate (0.5% higher) and **confined placental mosaicism.** Because chromosome mosaicism arises in somatic cells at a later stage in development, the abnormal cells may be confined to the placenta, the fetus, or both. Detection of mosaicism in placental tissue (CVS) is not indicative of abnormal karyotype in the fetus, the large majority of which are karyotypically normal. A second invasive procedure (usually amniocentesis) is necessary to provide reassurance to the parents after the detection of mosaicism through CVS.

3. E Children with DS have a 1% to 2% chance of developing acute lymphoblastic leukemia (20-fold greater than the general population). Interestingly **acquired** trisomy 21 is one of the most common chromosomal abnormalities seen in leukemia. A high incidence of seizure disorders (5% to 10%) is seen in children and adults with Alzheimer-like dementia who have DS. A high proportion of individuals with DS have thyroid dysfunction and hypothyroidism due to thyroid autoantibodies. Clinical recognition of hypothyroidism may be limited in DS, so routine screening is recommended. Atlantoaxial subluxation is a rare but serious complication of DS, associated with neurologic signs of spinal compression. It is likely related to the hyperextensibility of joints seen in DS.

Case 29

1. B CVS obtains only tissue sample from the chorionic villi. The possibility does exist that the karyotype of the chorionic villi and the fetus differ due to mosaicism, although the occurrence is very rare. In particular, confined placental mosaicism is when the trophoblastic cells in the placenta have undergone a nondisjunction, but the fetal cells have not. Cellular differentiation does not play a role in the development or the ability to detect DS, because the problem is at the germline. Nondisjunction during either meiosis I or II does not cause the presented scenario because we know that the chorionic villi contain a normal karyotype. The event causing the trisomy occurred after fertilization. If nondisjunction occurred during either meiotic event, the CVS would have detected it. If there was a paternal transmission of a genetic abnormality, this again should be detected by CVS because it would have affected the pregnancy at the time of fertilization, before the division of cells to form the placental tissue versus fetal tissue.

2. D During metaphase II, the chromosomes align along the equatorial plate and do not continue meiosis until fertilization. (Please review the text for the steps of meiosis.)

3. E The correct order for meiosis I is prophase I, metaphase I, anaphase I, and telophase I. Meiosis II follows with the same order, but there is no prophase II.

Case 30

1. E Manifesting heterozygous females for X-linked recessive disorders has been well documented, albeit rare. Homozygosity (two mutant alleles [one on each X chromosome]) can occur when there is an affected father and the mother is a carrier female or as a result of a new spontaneous mutation passed on by the mother (exceedingly rare). **Skewed X inactivation** is another explanation, although it is unlikely that the phenotype is as severe as with an affected male. There are several cases of Turner's syndrome girls with X-linked recessive conditions such as hemophilia A and DMD, who expressed the trait as X-linked dominant. The X chromosome involved in an autosomal translocation remains preferentially active, in order for the autosomal component of the derivative chromosome to maintain activity. So if the **breakpoint of the translocation disrupts a gene** on the X chromosome that remains preferentially active, a female can be affected with an X-linked recessive disorder. This concept has been used in **gene mapping.**

2. B Females with the Turner phenotype and signs of virilization should be screened for the presence of the Y chromosome. The karyotype may show various degrees of 45,X/46,XY mosaicism or the Y component may be detected by molecular methods such as FISH or PCR in cases of cryptic 45,X/46,XY mosaicism. These individuals with gonadal dysgenesis with a Y chromosome component are at an increased risk of developing a malignant germline tumor (gonadoblastoma). The recommendation is for removal of the gonads after reaching puberty because the gonads generally do not undergo malignant changes before then and their presence may aid in sexual development.

3. D Initial reports of individuals with sex chromosome abnormalities came from institutions for the mentally retarded or correction facilities for criminals. This selection bias contributed to descriptions of severe phenotypes, particularly for the XYY males and their "criminal Y chromosome," which have not held up in prospective studies of unselected populations. The phenotypes of

prenatally ascertained cases (amniocentesis and CVS) are not always the same as those for postnatally ascertained cases. For example, 45,X/46,XY cases diagnosed by amniocentesis secondary to screening due to maternal age are usually (90%) normal males at birth who would not have been otherwise recognized as abnormal, whereas postnatally diagnosed 45,X/46,XY have phenotypic abnormalities (usually ambiguous genitalia) 100% of the time! (That's why the study was ordered.) Imprinting has not been shown to play a role in phenotypic variability of sex chromosome abnormalities.

Case 31

1. E A karyotype with 69 chromosomes, or triploidy, is characteristic of partial moles. Studies using DNA polymorphism analysis have revealed that 46 of these chromosomes are always derived from the father, and the 23 remaining are maternally derived. This doubling of the paternal haploid set occurs either by duplication of the haploid sperm chromosome set or by fertilization of the egg by two sperm (dispermy). Unlike with complete moles, in partial moles, there is fetal development, but a liveborn infant almost never results. The rare cases of liveborn infants with triploidy have died within hours or a few days. Also important, partial moles have a very low malignant potential, unlike complete moles. Duplication of a male-derived chromosome set and empty ovum is one of the mechanisms invoked in complete moles. Failure to undergo second meiotic division in the developing ovum results in a diploid state, XX of all maternally derived cells. This is the explanation given for the formation of ovarian teratomas.

2. C **Mature cystic teratoma of the ovary** (also called **dermoid cyst**) is one of the most common benign ovarian tumors. Mature teratomas typically present in women between 20 and 30 years of age. These tumors are composed of mature ectoderm, mesoderm, and endoderm. Chromosome studies of these tumors reveal that the cells are of sole maternal origin, a process known as **parthenogenesis.** Ovarian teratomas appear to be the result of parthenogenetic development of the ovum that has not undergone the second meiotic division. Thus, these cells are diploid (46) and XX. 46,XX, paternally derived sets of chromosomes, is what is seen in 90% of complete moles (10% are 46,XY, again all paternally derived). Triploidy (69 chromosomes) is the karyotype seen in partial moles.

3. B Occasionally, a hyperthyroid state is seen in molar pregnancies; what has been called **gestational thyrotoxicosis.** There is abundant evidence that hCG is a weak thyrotropin (TSH) agonist. Marked elevations of hCG are a prominent feature of molar pregnancies. Excessive hCG secretion may cause hyperthyroidism in these patients. In normal pregnancy, when hCG levels are highest at 10 to 12 weeks of gestation, there is suppression of serum TSH levels, due to increases in free thyroxine (T_4) concentration. This situation can be exacerbated in the setting of a hydatiform mole. Unlike other causes of hyperthyroidism, the treatment consists of evacuation of the uterus, eliminating the source of thyroid stimulation. Care must be taken to avoid a thyroid storm during this transient phase.

Case 32

1. E There is a 50% chance that EY's children will receive the microdeletion. However, because his children would be receiving the mutation from their father, the affected children would have Prader-Willi syndrome and not Angelman's syndrome.

2. E In AD disorders, any affected parent can pass on the disorder. In AR disorders, two copies of a defective gene need to be inherited, one from each parent. In X-linked recessive disorders, only the male is affected while the female is the carrier. Although the inheritance pattern of Angelman's syndrome has similarities to mitochondrial inheritance, there is a key difference. In Angelman's syndrome, a father can theoretically pass on the disease. For example, if an affected father gives the chromosome 15 deletion to his daughter, she will have Prader-Willi syndrome. If the daughter then gives it to the grandchild, the grandchild will once again have Angelman's syndrome. This pattern would be impossible for mitochondrial inheritance.

3. B Beckwith-Wiedemann syndrome results from the overexpression of a growth factor gene, which is normally expressed only on paternal chromosome 11 and imprinted and inactivated on the maternal chromosome. This syndrome occurs when two copies of paternal chromosome 11 are inherited or if the imprinted maternal gene on chromosome 11 becomes activated. The symptoms of Beckwith-Wiedemann syndrome include large gestational size, large tongue, abdominal wall defects, and increased risk of Wilms' tumor (a renal cancer). DMD is an X-linked disorder, NF1 is an AD disorder, and CF and sickle-cell anemia are AR diseases.

Case 33

1. D HIV DNA is produced from its RNA genome while in the host cell cytoplasm by the reverse-transcriptase enzyme. HIV RNA, reverse-transcriptase, viral envelope, and integrase enzyme are all part of the invading HIV particle.

2. A HIV makes many of its proteins in a long continuous chain, which must be cleaved by the protease enzyme to create functional proteins needed for the assembly of new virus. Protease inhibitors bind to the active site of the protease enzyme, preventing its action. The integration of the HIV genetic material requires integrase while the reverse-transcriptase enzyme is needed to form the viral DNA copy from the original RNA genome.

3. D Mature HIV is composed of a lipid envelope, proteins, and an RNA genome. Because uracil is present only in RNA and thymine in DNA, both fluorescence-labeled uracil and amino acids can be detected in the new virus particles.

Case 34

1. B RNA splicing errors can result *from* nonsense and frameshift, but not vice versa. These mutations alter the splice donor and acceptor sites and can activate cryptic splice sites that compete with the normal splice sites, all at the end resulting in a nonfunctional or abnormal mRNA and protein. RNA is processed in the nucleus before transport into the cytoplasm. These processing steps include capping the 5′ end, polyadenylation of the 3′ end, and RNA splicing. Protein synthesis, which begins with binding of the 5′ cap by translation initiation factors, occurs in the cytoplasm. In RNA splicing, a lariat shape intermediate is formed in the primary RNA transcript at specific sites, snRNPs and the RNA form spliceosomes, and the intervening noncoding sequence is removed. The 5′ caps all contain a 7-methylguanylate.

2. B Nonsense mutations are associated with more severe damage than missense and silent mutations. A missense mutation is defined as a change in the amino acid, but it is a conservative change, meaning the new amino acid is similar in chemical structure as the one that was supposed to be encoded. A silent mutation is a mutation in which there is no change in the amino acid encoded but in which base change has occurred, typically in the third base position. A nonsense mutation refers to a change that results in an early stop codon. A frameshift mutation occurs when a change results in misreading of all codons downstream of the error and often results in an early stop codon and a truncated protein.

3. E Although the basic steps in protein synthesis are similar between prokaryotic and eukaryotic cells, they do differ in some aspects. In eukaryotes, the first AUG found is used as the start site while the Shine-Dalgarno sequence is important in the prokaryotic system in differentiating the start AUG from other AUG codons. The 30S and 50S ribosomal subunits are seen in prokaryotes, while 40S and 60S ribosomal subunits are found in eukaryotic cells. The *N*-formylmethionine is seen in prokaryotes and plain methionine is in eukaryotes. Protein synthesis is an energy-dependent process that requires ATP for tRNA charging and GTP for elongation and termination.

Case 35

1. D Point mutations occur in the genes encoding the variable regions of the heavy and light chains, and the resulting new codes are responsible for part of the diversity in antibody specificity that is seen. The diversity exists because of the somatic recombination (not homologous recombination) that occurs to bring a specific V, D, and J segment together, junctional diversity, and the different combinations created between different heavy and light chains. Homologous recombination is an exchange of genetic information between two homologous regions on a chromosome and typically occurs during meiosis. Deletion, translocation, and duplication are not known causes for antibody diversity.

2. D IgG is the only type of antibody that crosses the placenta and gives passive immunity to a fetus and newborn. By approximately 6 to 9 months, these antibodies are degraded. However, continued passive immunity may also be obtained through transmission of maternal IgG from breast milk. The other immunoglobulins are not able to pass through the placenta.

Case 36

1. E In α-thalassemia, there is an absence of Hgb F. Hgb H, a form of α-thalassemia in which three of the four α-globin genes are defective, is characterized by the precipitation of β-chain tetramers. Carriers of α-thalassemia are asymptomatic, without any anemia, whereas individuals with α-thalassemia minor have a mild microcytic anemia. β-Thalassemia is mainly caused by point mutations and is seen primarily in individuals of Mediterranean and African descent, whereas α-thalassemia is due to deletions and afflicts mostly Southeast Asians.

2. E Western blot analysis is not a method in gene mapping. It is a molecular biology technique whereby proteins are electrophoresed on a gel and then transferred to a filter. The filter is exposed to a labeled antibody specific to a protein of interest, and if this protein is present in the sample, it will be bound to the protein band in the gel. This technique is typically used to detect the presence of specific proteins in or expressed by a cell. The other methods are used in gene mapping. Positional cloning is an approach to cloning a gene based on its map position, which is determined by clues from linkage analysis. RFLP refers to inherited differences in sites for restriction enzymes that result in different lengths of fragments produced by specific restriction enzymes. These are used in gene mapping to link a gene or mutation to a genetic marker and allows for comparisons to determine whether someone carries a particular mutation. Somatic cell hybridization allows scientists to study the presence or absence of a particular gene by creating an immortal cell line amenable for study. The human cells of interest are combined in culture with somatic cells and are fused by adding Sendai virus or polyethylene glycol. These agents cause the fusion of membranes in the two cell types and after the resulting heterokaryons (a fusion of cells containing one of each cell type) can undergo cell division; the genetic information in the two cell types are mixed. These resulting clones can then be screened for the presence or absence of the gene of interest. Lastly, FISH is a process by which a fluorescent probe that identifies a particular gene or region of a chromosome is allowed to hybridize to chromosomes from the cells of interest to determine whether it is present.

3. D BPG is a by-product from the glycolysis pathway. It functions to decrease the affinity of O_2 from hemoglobin by binding to the deoxyhemoglobin, not the oxygenated form. It is not considered a cofactor because hemoglobin is not an enzyme. BPG binds weakly to Hgb F and therefore does not decrease the affinity of O_2 to Hgb F. This works in the maternal-fetal circulation because in the fetus there needs to be unloading of O_2 from the maternal circulation. Fetal hemoglobin needs to comparatively have a greater affinity for O_2 than maternal hemoglobin so that an exchange can be made in the placenta where the two circulations meet.

Case 37

1. E A nuclear family, with the affected individual and both parents, is necessary for **linkage analysis,** which can be done using **polymorphic markers flanking the gene locus.** Using this principle, the disease-causing allele can be determined and prenatal testing pos-

sible by means of CVS or amniocentesis. This technique has been used successfully for many genetic diseases in which there is no direct DNA testing but gene locus is known. Second-trimester US is of no use in the prenatal diagnosis of A-T, because there are no specific findings in affected fetuses that can be seen by US. AFP in amniotic fluid has been used successfully in the detection of NTDs, along with acetylcholinesterase, both of which are elevated in the presence of open NTDs. Chromosomal breakage is an interesting option for the antenatal diagnosis of A-T when there is no DNA testing, but unfortunately, it has not been reliable enough.

2. D Several rare AR conditions have a relatively high incidence in certain populations. This is likely the result of a combination of a **founder effect,** and social, religious, or geographic isolation. The founder effect is where by chance, one or two of the original founders of the community had the mutant allele and passed it on to a large number of his or her descendants. Rare AR disorders have been associated with increased frequency of consanguinity. However, in these cases, the mutation is often "private" to that particular family. The **Hardy-Weinberg principle** states that the frequency of each genotype stays unchanged or in *equilibrium* in subsequent generations. **Heterozygote advantage** is a plausible explanation for the relatively high frequency of a serious AR disorder in large populations. Good examples of heterozygote advantage are sickle-cell anemia and β-thalassemia and the relative advantage of heterozygous (carriers) against malaria.

Case 38

1. B G1 is known to vary most between cell types and accounts for the differences in doubling time between cell types. G0, or quiescence, refers to cells not in the cell cycle. Typically, the S phase lasts 20 hours, G2 lasts 3 hours, and M phase lasts 1 hour for most cell types.

2. A The presence of Okazaki's fragments causes a block in the S phase and progression through S does not occur until they are all cleared. An increase in p53 leads to a block in G1/S. Rb acts to block the cell cycle by binding to E2F, thereby preventing its action. p27 binds to cyclin-Cdk to prevent their activity. Cyclins bind to Cdk and the active cyclin-Cdk complexes phosphorylate downstream targets.

Case 39

1. A Only toxoplasmosis is caused by the protozoan *Toxoplasma gondii.* Rubella is part of the togavirus family made up of enveloped RNA viruses. CMV and HSV are enveloped linear dsDNA viruses and are members of the herpesvirus family. Syphilis is caused by the spirochete *Treponema pallidum.*

2. E The distinctive presentation of rhinitis, rash on the palms and soles, and poor feeding is consistent with congenital syphilis. This diagnosis is made definitively by dark-field microscopy. As an older infant, other abnormalities will likely become apparent as well, including bone and/or joint pain, mental retardation, and vision and/or hearing loss. Rubella can be diagnosed by the detection of rubella-specific IgM antibodies in the infant, isolation of the virus from nasopharyngeal or urine specimens, or the persistence of rubella IgG after 8 to 12 months. HSV diagnosis is made by culturing samples from vesicles, urine, or the nasopharynx. The diagnosis of CMV can be made by neonatal urine culture or serum antibody titer.

3. A Although infection generally presents with flulike symptoms in a healthy adult, the symptoms can be much more severe in an immunocompromised individual. This intracellular parasite can invade the CNS and patients present with fever, mental status changes, lethargy, headache, seizures, and focal neurologic findings. CT scan is significant for multiple ring-enhancing lesions and cerebral edema. The source of the infection can be from the soil, undercooked meat, or cat feces, or it can be due to reactivation of oocytes in an immunocompromised host.

Case 40

1. B **DiGeorge's syndrome** occurs because third and fourth pharyngeal pouches fail to differentiate into the thymus and the parathyroid glands. The facial abnormalities are the result of alterations in the development of the first arch. It is now known that DiGeorge's and velocardiofacial syndrome (VCFS) are different ends of the spectrum of the same entity. The most common features of VCFS are cleft palate, heart defects, characteristic facial appearance, minor learning problems, and speech and feeding problems. VCFS/DiGeorge's is one of the most common genetic syndromes. Most cases are caused by **a microdeletion of chromosome 22q.**

2. E Isolated cleft lip with or without cleft palate is a classic example of **MFI**, which is explained by the liability/threshold model. A multifactorial trait is exhibited if the liability surpasses the threshold. The recurrence risks for MFI are influenced by the disease severity, the degree of relationship to the index case, the number of affected close relatives, and the sex of the index case if there is a higher incidence of the disorder in one particular sex. Cleft lip results from failure of mesenchymal masses in the medial nasal and maxillary prominence to merge between 4 and 8 weeks of development. **Chromosomal abnormalities and single-gene defects** account for a small part of children with cleft lip and palate. **Teratogenic exposures** including antiepileptics, cigarette smoking, and large amounts of ethanol consumption have been associated with an increased risk of cleft lip and palate.

3. E Isolated cleft palate is considered a separate entity from cleft lip or cleft lip and palate. It occurs as a result of failure of the mesenchymal masses in the palatine processes to meet and fuse, because of the abnormal migration of the neural crest cell from the first arch. Fusion of the palate begins at about 8 weeks and is completed by 12 weeks. Microdeletions of chromosome 22q (VCFS syndrome) frequently have cleft palate as a feature. This is an AD disorder, although most affected individuals are the product of de novo deletions. Folate acid deficiency and/or enzymatic defects in the folate acid pathway have been associated with an increase risk of cleft lip and palate and isolated cleft palate.

Case 41

1. C Only organs arising from the ectoderm (CNS, face, ears, eyes) seem to be affected in this patient. The mesoderm layer gives rise to the musculoskeletal, cardiovascular, and genitourinary systems, whereas the endoderm forms the GI and respiratory tracts.

2. B The major birth defect associated with thalidomide is deformity of the long bones, resulting in amelia or meromelia (total or partial absence of the extremities). Isotretinoin causes abnormal ear development, cleft palate, and NTDs/heart defects. Lithium has been implicated in heart malformations (Ebstein's anomaly), whereas alcohol causes FAS (growth retardation, facial dysmorphisms, mental retardation, and heart defects). DES is a synthetic estrogen that has been linked to genitourinary cancer and malformations in young women who were exposed in utero.

3. E The formation of the embryonic germ layers occurs during gastrulation that starts with the appearance of the primitive streak on the epiblast and ends with the invagination of the epiblast cells to form the endoderm and mesoderm. Cleavage represents a series of cell divisions without an increase in overall size that characterizes early development of the embryo. Compaction is the process by which blastomeres form a compact ball of cells during the cleavage process.

Case 42

1. B Periconceptional (from before conception to at least 10 to 12 weeks of gestation) ingestion of high-dose folic acid (4 mg) has been shown to reduce the recurrence of NTDs in RCTs. First occurrence of NTDs is reduced by the periconceptional intake of 0.4 mg of folic acid. Women of reproductive age exposed to the possibility of pregnancy should be encouraged to take adequate amounts of folic acid, because more than half of pregnancies in the United States are planned. Consumption of large amounts of alcohol in pregnancy may lead to the FAS, which is characterized by mild mental retardation and distinctive facial features, not NTDs. Heavy doses of ionizing radiation, far greater than those from x-ray exposure, have been associated with microcephaly and ocular defects.

2. C Like most other malformations involving a single organ (e.g., VSD and cleft lip), most NTDs show an MFI, implying an interaction of many genes with the environment. Other causes are more rare but well established as causes of NTDs such as **teratogens** (valproic acid), **vitamin deficiency** (coal-mine regions of Wales before dietary supplementation of folic acid), **single-gene defects** (Meckel's syndrome AR characterized by polydactyly, encephalocele, and polycystic kidneys), and **chromosomal abnormalities** (trisomy 13 and trisomy 18).

3. E **Valproic acid** is a well-established teratogen, increasing the risk of NTDs 10- to 20-fold over background risk (6%) when administered during the first trimester of pregnancy. Most of the defects occur during the third and fourth week of development (5 to 6 weeks of LMP). Earlier exposures (1 to 2 weeks of development) either are associated with early pregnancy loss or are of no consequence to the fetus (**all-or-nothing phenomenon**). Other **anticonvulsants** are also associated with an increased risk of NTDs (carbamazepine) and minor congenital anomalies (phenytoin) but to a much smaller degree than valproic acid.

Case 43

1. B DiGeorge's syndrome is caused by abnormal development of the third and fourth pharyngeal pouches that give rise to the thymus and the parathyroid glands. The second pharyngeal arch develops into the stapes and hyoid bones, as well as the muscles facial expression. The third arch forms the remainder of the hyoid bone and the stylopharyngeus muscle. The first cleft develops into the external auditory meatus. The second aortic arch forms the hyoid and stapedial arteries, and the third aortic arch creates the common carotid, external carotid, and part of the internal carotid arteries. The fifth pharyngeal pouch differentiates into the ultimo-branchial body that eventually becomes the parafollicular or C-cells of the thyroid.

2. C These bones are mostly formed by the first pharyngeal arch and are derived from embryologic mesodermal cells. The cells of the pharyngeal cleft are composed of ectoderm, and those of the pharyngeal pouch are of endodermal origin.

3. E The cricothyroid muscle is derived from the fourth pharyngeal arch and is the only intrinsic muscle of the larynx not produced by the sixth arch. It is supplied by the superior laryngeal nerve, while all muscles of the sixth arch are innervated by the recurrent laryngeal nerve. Recurrent laryngeal nerve dysfunction (from trauma or mass lesion) is the most common cause of vocal cord paralysis and hoarseness.

Case 44

1. B This abnormal process will produce a persistent truncus arteriosus, which overrides both ventricles and eventually branches into the aorta and pulmonary artery. The transposition of the great vessels arises when the conotruncal septum descends straight down instead of in a spiral pattern. The result is that the aorta arises from the right ventricle while the pulmonary artery originates from the left ventricle. Valvular stenosis is caused by either the fusion of the thickened valves or a narrowed outflow tract. Tetralogy of Fallot is caused by the anterior displacement of the conotruncal septum and results in an overriding aorta, pulmonary stenosis, VSD, and right ventricle hypertrophy. Dextrocardia occurs when the cardiac loop forms on the opposite side and results in the eventual placement of the heart in the right side of the thorax.

2. C PGE_1 is an arachidonic acid (AA) derivative that relaxes ductal smooth muscle and causes the dilation of the ductus arteriosus. Both indomethacin and ibuprofen are NSAIDs that decrease prostaglandin production and are used to close a PDA. Dexamethasone is a glucocorticoid, and although TXA_2 is also an AA product, it causes platelet aggregation and increased vascular tone.

3. B The ostium secundum is the opening in the septum secundum through which blood can flow from the right to the left atrium. The septum primum is adjacent to the septum secundum and acts as a valve for the foramen ovale. The condition described is caused by the premature closing of the foramen ovale by the fusion of the septum primum and the septum secundum. This condition usually results in death soon after birth. Absence of the atrial septum or inadequate formation of the septum secundum would result in increased blood flow from the right atrium to the left atrium. Failure of the endocardial cushions to fuse can also result in a septal defect or a persistent atrioventricular canal.

Case 45

1. B RDS, also known as **hyaline membrane disease,** is caused by inadequate secretion of surfactant at the lung surface in premature infants. Surfactant is a phospholipid-rich fluid that acts to prevent the formation of high surface tension at the alveoli surface. Shortly after the syndrome begins, the alveoli are frequently covered with a layer of hyaline membrane and a high-protein fluid. The use of synthetic surfactant and glucocorticoid treatment to stimulate the production of surfactant have contributed to the increased survival of premature babies.

2. A The epithelium of the lung is derived from the endodermal germ layer, as are other structures that grow from the foregut (e.g., stomach, liver, pancreas, and intestines) and hindgut (e.g., intestines and bladder). The heart, kidney, and spleen are of mesodermal origin, and the lens of the eye is derived from the ectodermal germ layer.

3. C The muscles of the larynx are derived from the fourth and sixth pharyngeal arches. The fourth pharyngeal pouch forms the superior parathyroid gland. There is no sixth pharyngeal pouch. The first pharyngeal cleft gives rise to the external auditory meatus. The third pharyngeal pouch creates the thymus and the inferior parathyroid gland, and the third pharyngeal arch forms the hyoid bone and stylopharyngeus muscle.

Case 46

1. C Elevations in MSAFP are seen in open **NTDs,** as well as **ventral abdominal wall defects** such as gastroschisis and omphalocele. Because in gastroschisis, there is no sac that contains the intestinal contents, the elevations in AFP tend to be higher than those seen in omphaloceles. Duodenal atresia, as well as any other obstruction of the upper GI tract, is associated with polyhydramnios. There is a characteristic "double bubble" caused by the dilation of the stomach and proximal duodenum that can be seen in both prenatal US and postnatal x-ray. Duodenal atresia is associated with DS in 30% of cases. Annular pancreas is rare and causes obstruction of the GI tract. Congenital ileal diverticulum (Meckel's diverticulum) is a remnant of the yolk sac. They are common and may mimic appendicitis or ulcerate and bleed. In congenital megacolon or Hirschsprung's disease, a part of the colon is dilated as a result of the absence of autonomic ganglion.

2. B Esophageal atresia is associated with **tracheoesophageal fistula in 85% of the cases.** The x-rays typically show a stop of the nasogastric tube at the level of the esophagus, but there is air in the stomach (there is no air in the stomach in isolated esophageal atresia). There is an incomplete separation of the esophagus from the laryngotracheal tube, because of the deviation of the tracheoesophageal septum into a posterior direction. Failure of recanalization or incomplete recanalization at any point in the digestive tract results in atresia or stenosis, respectively. Congenital megacolon is caused by failure of migration of the neural crest cells to the wall of the colon.

3. B The midgut migrates into the proximal portion of the umbilical cord during the sixth week. This is a result of the restricted space inside the abdomen, which is due to the relatively large liver undergoing hematopoiesis and the rapid growth of the midgut. At around the tenth week, there is a normal return to the abdomen of the intestines. Before the intestines return to the abdomen, a 90-degree counterclockwise rotation occurs. The extraembryonic portion of the **allantois** degenerates in the second month. Its intraembryonic portion runs from the apex of the bladder to the umbilicus and involutes into a thick tubular structure, the **urachus.** After birth, the urachus becomes a fibrous band, the median umbilical ligament.

Case 47

1. B Prolonged rupture of the membranes at mid gestation or earlier, causing chronic leakage of amniotic fluid and hence severe oligohydramnios, may lead to limb-positioning defects, abnormal facies, and pulmonary hypoplasia. This is referred to as the **oligohydramnios sequence.** Whatever the cause, the absence of amniotic fluid has a profound impact on the developing fetus. CDH is associated with pulmonary hypoplasia because of the compression from the abdominal viscera occupying the thoracic cavity. However the amniotic fluid is normal or increased, so there are no other manifestations of fetal compression. In unilateral renal agenesis, the remaining kidney generally has normal function because there are normal amounts of amniotic fluid. Thanatophoric dysplasia is a lethal form of dwarfism, with marked narrowing of the chest, leading to pulmonary hypoplasia and respiratory insufficiency. There is an intrinsic bone abnormality, not a deformation,

caused by mutations in the gene encoding fibroblast growth factor receptor-3 (FGFR3). It is AD and is caused by new mutations.

2. D Prolonged rupture of membranes is by far the most common cause of oligohydramnios in pregnancy. The presence of amniotic fluid in the vagina, on gross examination and confirmed by placing the sample on a microscopic slide, air drying, and visualization of a "ferning" pattern, is diagnostic. US examination in rupture of membranes may demonstrate no amniotic fluid, but the fetal bladder and kidneys should be seen. The differentiation of these two entities is crucial, Because BRA is invariably lethal, whereas prolonged rupture of the membranes is not, and its prognosis is largely related to the gestational age at its occurrence and the degree of amniotic fluid reduction. Other causes of absence of amniotic fluid include severe dysplastic kidneys and complete urinary obstruction

3. C The composition of amniotic fluid varies with gestational age. Initially, most of the amniotic fluid comes from diffusion of interstitial fluid across the amniochorionic membrane. Later, there is diffusion of fluid from blood in the intervillous space of the placenta. Urine production by the fetal kidneys begins at 11 weeks. After 16 to 18 weeks, fetal urine accounts for more than 98% of the amniotic fluid. Amniotic fluid is swallowed and then absorbed by the fetuses respiratory and digestive systems and then enters into the fetal circulation, where it crosses the placenta into the maternal bloodstream. Alterations at any of these levels result in alterations of the amniotic fluid volume. Copious maternal water intake may result in a modest transient increase in amniotic fluid volume.

4. E Exstrophy of the bladder is a severe anomaly that occurs predominantly in males, where the trigone and the ureteric orifices are exposed through the lower abdominal wall. The defect involves the anterior abdominal wall and the anterior wall of the bladder and is caused by failure of the mesenchymal cells to migrate between the ectoderm of the abdomen and the cloaca during the fourth week. Divisions of the metanephric diverticulum (ureteric bud) give rise to duplications of the urinary tract, which are fairly common. Incomplete division results in a divided kidney with a bifid ureter. Complete division results in a double kidney with a bifid or separate ureter. The urachus is a thick fibrous cord extending from the apex of the bladder to the umbilicus, which is derived from the allantois, a vestigial structure. Patency of the urachus (urachal fistula) causes dribbling of urine at the umbilicus, not bladder exstrophy.

Index

Index note: page references with an *f* or *t* indicate a figure or table on that page.